T0192929

18
LEVERS
FOR
HIGH-IMPACT
PERFORMANCE
IMPROVEMENT

ACHE Management Series Editorial Board

Lisa Piercey, MD, FACHE, Chairman
West Tennessee Healthcare

Daniel L. Avosso, MD, FACHE
The Regional Medical Center of Orangeburg and Calhoun Counties

Jeremy S. Bradshaw, FACHE
MountainView Hospital

Cassandra S. Crowal, FACHE
MidState Medical Center

Alison Flynn Gaffney, FACHE
Nexera, Inc., and GNYHA Services, Inc.

Mona E. Miliner, FACHE
University of Cincinnati

Philip R. Pullum
Real Radiology, LLC

Angela Rivera
CTG Health Solutions

Atefeh Samadi-niya, MD, DHA, FACHE
IRACA Solutions, Inc.

Jason A. Spring, FACHE
Kalispell Regional Healthcare System

David R. Steinmann, FACHE
Mercy Hospital Lebanon

Col Andrea Vinyard
HQ Air Education and Training Command

18

LEVERS
FOR
HIGH-IMPACT
PERFORMANCE
IMPROVEMENT

How
Healthcare
Organizations
Can Accelerate
Change and
Sustain Results

Gary M. Auton

ACHE Management Series

Your board, staff, or clients may also benefit from this book's insight. For information on quantity discounts, contact the Health Administration Press Marketing Manager at (312) 424-9450.

This publication is intended to provide accurate and authoritative information in regard to the subject matter covered. It is sold, or otherwise provided, with the understanding that the publisher is not engaged in rendering professional services. If professional advice or other expert assistance is required, the services of a competent professional should be sought.

The statements and opinions contained in this book are strictly those of the author and do not represent the official positions of the American College of Healthcare Executives or the Foundation of the American College of Healthcare Executives.

Copyright © 2018 by the Foundation of the American College of Healthcare Executives. Printed in the United States of America. All rights reserved. This book or parts thereof may not be reproduced in any form without written permission of the publisher.

22   21   20   19   18   5   4   3   2   1

Library of Congress Cataloging-in-Publication Data
Names: Auton, Gary M., author.
Title: 18 levers for high-impact performance improvement : how healthcare
   organizations can accelerate change and sustain results / Gary M. Auton.
Other titles: Eighteen levers for high-impact performance improvement
Description: Chicago, IL : Health Administration Press, [2018] | Series:
   HAP/ACHE management series | Includes bibliographical references. |
   Identifiers: LCCN 2018001852 (print) | LCCN 2018006838 (ebook) | ISBN
   9781567939965 (ebook) | ISBN 9781567939972 (xml) | ISBN 9781567939989
   (epub) | ISBN 9781567939996 (mobi) | ISBN 9781567939958 (alk. paper)
Subjects: LCSH: Medical care—Quality control. | Medicine—Practice—Finance.
   | Medical offices—Management. | Medical care—Evaluation.
Classification: LCC RA399.A1 (ebook) | LCC RA399.A1 A98 2018 (print) | DDC
   362.1068/1—dc23
LC record available at https://lccn.loc.gov/2018001852

The paper used in this publication meets the minimum requirements of American National Standard for Information Sciences—Permanence of Paper for Printed Library Materials, ANSI Z39.48-1984. ∞ ™

Acquisitions editor: Jennette McClain; Project manager: Joyce Dunne; Cover designer: Brad Norr; Layout: PerfecType

Found an error or a typo? We want to know! Please e-mail it to hapbooks@ache.org, mentioning the book's title and putting "Book Error" in the subject line.

For photocopying and copyright information, please contact Copyright Clearance Center at www.copyright.com or at (978) 750-8400.

Health Administration Press
A division of the Foundation of the American
   College of Healthcare Executives
300 S. Riverside Plaza, Suite 1900
Chicago, IL 60606-6698
(312) 424-2800

Brief Contents

Acknowledgments   xiii

Introduction   xv

Part I   **Performance Acceleration in Healthcare Organizations**

Chapter 1   The Emerging Healthcare Business Model   3

Chapter 2   Assessing the Starting Point   19

Chapter 3   A New Framework for Healthcare Performance Improvement   39

Part II   **Healthcare Performance Improvement Levers**

Chapter 4   Improving Processes and Facilities   59

Chapter 5   Aligning Resources with Demand   107

Chapter 6   Leveraging the System   157

Chapter 7   Optimizing Nonlabor Expenses   183

Chapter 8   Improving Quality and Clinical Utilization   197

Chapter 9   Building Revenues   223

Chapter 10   Optimizing the Service Portfolio   255

Part III   **Design, Implementation, and Performance Monitoring**

Chapter 11   Structure and Process for Performance Improvement   281

Chapter 12   Leading Implementation   305

Chapter 13   Three Disciplines for Holding the Gains   327

*Appendix A: Organizational Assessment Template
for Performance Improvement Competencies*   359
*Appendix B: The 18 Performance Improvement Levers
for Healthcare Systems*   367
*Appendix C: Application of Improvement Levers
by Functional Area*   393
References   397
About the Author   401

Detailed Contents

Acknowledgments   xiii

Introduction   xv

**Part I   Performance Acceleration in Healthcare
             Organizations**

Chapter 1   The Emerging Healthcare Business Model   3

            How Healthcare's Business Model
               Is Evolving   4

            Operational Challenges in the
               New Healthcare Environment   7

            Implications for Performance Improvement   16

Chapter 2   Assessing the Starting Point   19

            Performance Improvement Leadership   19

            Workforce Engagement   22

            Consumer Engagement   25

            Physician Engagement   26

            Data-Driven Management   30

            Prelaunch Organizational Assessment   31

            Identification of Improvement
               Opportunities and Goal Setting   33

Chapter 3   A New Framework for Healthcare
            Performance Improvement   39

            Issues in Health System Performance
               Improvement   43

A New Performance Improvement
    Framework   44

Change Levers   48

Performance Levers and Health System
    Functions   49

System-Level Gap Closure Plan   50

Seven Performance Improvement Categories 55

Part II   Healthcare Performance Improvement Levers

Chapter 4   Improving Processes and Facilities   59

Lever 1: Process Improvement   60

Case Example: Process Improvement—
    Surgical Room Turnover   67

Lever 2: Structural Process Improvement   83

Case Example: Cross-Functional Process
    Improvement   89

Lever 3: Facility Optimization   95

Chapter 5   Aligning Resources with Demand   107

Labor Productivity Management   108

Demand Matching   110

Case Example: Predictive Modeling for
    Acute Care Nursing   113

Work Measurement and Activity Analysis 116

Lever 4: Demand Smoothing   118

Case Example: Surgical Block Scheduling 122

Lever 5: Demand Regrouping   125

Lever 6: Role and Team Redesign   130

Case Example: Role Design in an
    Emergency Department   136

Lever 7: Dynamic Staffing   146

Case Example: Seasonal Staffing Plan   154

Chapter 6   Leveraging the System   157

    Lever 8: Management Restructuring   159

    Lever 9: System Rationalization   165

    Lever 10: Service Redeployment   173

    Case Example: Redeploying
        Support Services   178

Chapter 7   Optimizing Nonlabor Expenses   183

    Supply Strategies   184

    Strategies Related to Medical Devices   186

    Tactics for Managing Pharmaceutical
        Expenses   187

    Lever 11: Nonlabor Optimization   189

    Supply Chain Improvement   189

Chapter 8   Improving Quality and Clinical Utilization   197

    Lever 12: Off-Quality Improvement   201

    Lever 13: Clinical Utilization
        Improvement   206

    Case Example: Clinical Utilization
        Improvement Team   217

Chapter 9   Building Revenues   223

    High-Growth Health Systems   225

    Lever 14: Demand Growth   228

    Case Example: Growing Home
        Health Services   233

    Growth as a Productivity Lever   237

    Lever 15: Revenue Optimization   237

Chapter 10   Optimizing the Service Portfolio   255

    Portfolio Review   257

    Portfolio Collaborative Teams   264

    Nonclinical Portfolio Review   265

Lever 16: Service Outsourcing   270

Lever 17: Service Divestment   273

Lever 18: Continuum Realignment   274

Part III   **Design, Implementation, and Performance Monitoring**

Chapter 11   Structure and Process for Performance Improvement   281

    Performance Improvement Collaborative Teams   282

    The Redesign Phase   284

    The Collaborative Team Process   288

    Case Example: Performance Improvement Plan for Pharmacy Services   298

Chapter 12   Leading Implementation   305

    Steering Committee Presentation and Review   307

    Implementation Teams   314

    Case Example: Organizing for Implementation   319

    Addressing Implementation Issues   320

Chapter 13   Three Disciplines for Holding the Gains   327

    Labor Performance Management System   327

    Supply Chain Value Analysis   347

    Case Example: Implementing a Value Analysis Team Structure and Process   351

    Growth and Strategy   355

    Key Takeaways for High-Impact Performance Improvement   357

Appendix A: Organizational Assessment Template for Performance Improvement Competencies   359

Appendix B: The 18 Performance Improvement Levers for Healthcare Systems   367

Appendix C: Application of Improvement Levers by Functional Area   393

References   397

About the Author   401

Acknowledgments

THE AUTHOR WOULD like to thank all the members of Galloway Consulting for their contributions to and support in the development of this book. Additionally, special thanks are extended to the following individuals, who generously provided external peer review and feedback: Rhonda M. Anderson, DNSc, RN, LFACHE, FAAN, of RMA Consulting; Linda Q. Everett, PhD, RN, NEA-BC, FAAN, an adjunct professor in the School of Nursing at Indiana University and a leadership consultant; and Rita Turley, RN, president of Turley Consulting and past president of the American Organization of Nurse Executives.

Acknowledgments

Introduction

"Health care is the most difficult, chaotic and complex industry to manage today."

—Peter Drucker

DRUCKER'S OBSERVATION, ABOVE, was written more than two decades ago, but it is even more relevant today. Although healthcare has always been organic and somewhat volatile, the industry is now experiencing a revolution. The US healthcare system continues to pose one of the nation's greatest domestic challenges as, confronted with spiraling costs and suboptimal quality and service outcomes, healthcare consumers and payers are clamoring for increased transparency and enhanced service value at reduced cost.

The move to value-based reimbursement is altering the structure and focus of healthcare organizations. This emerging business model compels providers to produce demonstrated, measurable results for the services they provide, delivered in a manner that increases service access and enhances patient engagement. All of these goals must be accomplished at diminished reimbursement levels.

At the epicenter of the change are health systems and the physicians, executives, and managers who lead them. The pressure is on these leaders to continuously improve services, streamline costs, and preserve operating margins. That said, overcoming the daily challenges to reduce operating expenses, advance service quality, and improve clinical quality outcomes is not possible unless the organization has sustained revenue growth and margins necessary for reinvestment in facilities, equipment, and other capital outlays.

For purposes of discussion in this book, the term *health system* refers to large, multientity healthcare organizations that provide services along the care continuum. Regional health systems may include multiple acute care hospitals, outpatient services, physician practices, post-acute care services, and other programs.

Every sea change demands strong leadership and a winning game plan to achieve enduring success. That game plan is performance improvement (PI). More than ever, health system leaders need stringent operating disciplines and effective improvement strategies to steer their organizations through an increasingly uncertain and complex environment.

Fad diets come and go, and most prove ineffective in the long term. Often, healthcare leaders view emerging PI models the same way. This perception is not without basis. For the past 30 years, the industry has seen numerous improvement philosophies, and approaches come and go. But even past improvement philosophies offer valid principles and lessons that can be applied effectively to healthcare organizations today.

PREMISES OF THIS BOOK

The purpose of this book is to serve as a resource and guide for healthcare leaders who are tasked with improving financial performance in their organizations. The principles in this book are a result of work with hundreds of hospitals and health systems across the country over more than 30 years. This work is centered on applying systems engineering principles and methods to improve organizational performance and restore operating margins and profitability.

The framework at the core of this model is built on a taxonomy of 18 improvement "levers" deployed at different levels of an organization. The framework is not intended to replace Lean, Six Sigma, or other PI approaches. Rather, it is a prioritizing structure by which to consistently apply PI principles and tools to those areas that have the highest impact on the patient experience, the quality of care outcomes, and healthcare costs. Using the rapid-cycle collaborative team process, organizations can further accelerate improvement by increasing speed to benefit.

The model and approaches in this book are based on three premises.

Premise 1: The changing business of healthcare requires performance improvement interventions that are faster, broader, and more strategic than those adopted in the past.

- Slow, incremental improvement is insufficient for most organizations to overcome the financial challenges they face.
- The traditional operational levers of labor productivity, supply, and revenue cycle improvements, while important, do not alone offset reimbursement and volume declines.
- Performance improvement must increasingly focus on long-term, high-impact areas, including clinical utilization, management restructuring, and systems rationalization.
- Building the new, patient-centric continuum of care requires a fundamental restructuring of the healthcare system. Some components will require heavy investment while investment in other components declines. To do so well, organizations need effective portfolio management processes and disciplines.

Premise 2: Most health systems are organized and structured in a similar manner; consequently, they share similar, predictable operational challenges.

- Most operational challenges in a health system are artifacts of structural issues of compartmentalization and complex cross-functional processes.

- Depending on the department or function, a short list of interventions provides most of the operational improvement opportunity.
- Leaders should prioritize and structure PI initiatives on the basis of these short lists.

Premise 3: Most performance improvement initiatives fall short of expectations not from a lack of skills, effort, structure, or tools but from an absence of prioritization and alignment.

- Health system leaders are often sidetracked by competing priorities, making the speedy and purposeful execution and sustained momentum of large-scale improvement initiatives difficult.
- Many organizations make substantial investments in PI staffing, training, and other resources but often fail to deploy these resources to areas and issues that provide the highest returns.
- Improvement initiatives often pay undue attention to assessing current processes and operational issues. This focus prolongs the time needed to identify and implement improvements and redesigned systems.
- The most difficult PI goals to achieve are implementation and sustainability. This issue often reflects a culture that lacks alignment and accountability.

Has the healthcare revolution finally arrived? That remains to be seen, but today's healthcare arena promises to be challenging and exciting for healthcare leaders.

PART I

Performance Acceleration in Healthcare Organizations

CHAPTER 1

The Emerging Healthcare Business Model

COMPELLED BY THE urgency to rein in costs and improve quality and access, US health policymakers and consumers are demanding greater accountability and demonstrated value from healthcare providers. These forces are fundamentally altering how care is financed and delivered, in turn transforming the business of healthcare delivery.

Historically, healthcare organizations succeeded by performing more and more services to an increasing number of patients. Hospitals and health systems leveraged their brand and expanded services to attract more patients. Revenues grew with increases in patient volumes. When revenues exceeded operating costs, healthcare organizations could reinvest gains into equipment and facilities, invest in human capital, and build brand recognition in the markets they served. Absent a disruption to this cycle—a drop in patient volumes, uncontrolled operating expenses, or adverse quality events—healthcare providers could continue to prosper.

Over time, the old volume-driven, fee-for-service model has resulted in medical cost growth that has far outpaced general inflation. Medical consumers, including patients, health plans, and employer groups, have paid increasingly higher costs with limited means to measure outcomes and value. Recent healthcare policy reform, new payer strategies, and the forces of consumerism are poised to bring greater information and control to consumers while requiring greater provider accountability and transparency than has been seen in healthcare in the past. These forces represent a fundamental challenge to the traditional healthcare business model.

HOW HEALTHCARE'S BUSINESS MODEL IS EVOLVING

Faced with these challenges, healthcare providers must adapt to this new environment by adopting a new success model. The emerging business model in healthcare (exhibit 1.1) is based on the requirement of providers to produce demonstrated, measurable results for the services they provide at a cost that is affordable to consumers.

The model is made up of three primary components: results, revenue, and margin, as discussed in the following paragraphs.

Exhibit 1.1: The Emerging Business Model for Healthcare Organizations

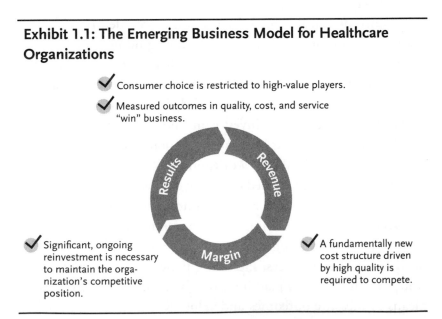

✔ Consumer choice is restricted to high-value players.

✔ Measured outcomes in quality, cost, and service "win" business.

✔ Significant, ongoing reinvestment is necessary to maintain the organization's competitive position.

✔ A fundamentally new cost structure driven by high quality is required to compete.

Results

Providers must produce consistent results that meet the needs of healthcare consumers. In this context, results are the outcomes and value a healthcare entity or practitioner delivers to the patients served. These outcomes are a composite of three performance dimensions, which align with the Triple Aim of the Institute for Healthcare Improvement as explained by Berwick, Nolan, and Whittington (2008):

- *Clinical quality.* The organization provides high-quality, evidence-based clinical services that ensure patient safety and consistently achieve high-quality outcomes.
- *Service quality.* The organization provides excellent customer service through streamlined, patient-centric processes that facilitate access and efficient care that is reflected in high patient satisfaction scores.
- *Cost performance.* The organization provides cost-effective care that is market competitive and produces high value to patients and the communities served.

Increasingly, providers are required to track multiple metrics along these performance dimensions and share results with patients, payers, and the public. Armed with this information, consumers will increasingly migrate to high-value providers. This trend will, in turn, create mandates for competing providers to improve their performance.

Revenue

Fee-for-service reimbursement for healthcare services represents a shrinking portion of payments for those services. Increasingly, a healthcare organization's revenues will be based on the results they produce. A variety of payment programs now reward providers on the basis of their performance, including the following:

- *Medicare accountable care organizations (ACOs)* are intended to drive the coordination of care for Medicare patients, particularly those with chronic conditions. ACO payments include bundled payments that combine hospital and physician service remuneration. ACOs share in the savings that accrue through the program (CMS 2017a).
- *Medicare's Hospital Value-Based Purchasing program* withholds a portion of participating hospitals' acute care reimbursement and rewards or penalizes organizations on the basis of their quartile ranking in multiple clinical and service performance measures (CMS 2017d; AHRQ 2017).
- *Case- or episode-based payment arrangements* have been established for high-volume, high-cost services such as joint replacement surgery and usually bundle the hospital and physician professional fee. Providers are financially motivated to provide care at lowered costs.
- *Direct contracting mechanisms* are used by many large employers to obtain care for their employees. These arrangements usually have negotiated pricing, including case-based payment.
- *Capitation* sets a fixed amount that healthcare organizations are paid per month to provide for the total healthcare needs of patients.

Each of these payment methodologies places greater financial risk on providers than in the past and requires organizations to adopt new systems and learn new competencies to manage costs and improve quality performance. Hospitals and physicians must work together to coordinate and deliver high-quality, cost-effective care for patients. For low-performing health systems, payment reform will result in anemic or declining revenues for facility and professional services.

Margin

Organizations must generate operating margins for reinvestment in medical technologies, information systems, facilities, and new programs and services. Organizations that cannot generate sufficient operating margins are unable to pursue new markets, improve existing services, or enhance the organization's brand in the community.

As reimbursement pressures build, organizations will need to focus increased attention on reducing operating expenses to maintain sufficient margins. The new reimbursement systems will require new or reimagined operating structures that deliver quality care at substantially reduced costs. For most providers, this expectation creates significant disruption to current health system organization and management.

OPERATIONAL CHALLENGES IN THE NEW HEALTHCARE ENVIRONMENT

The emerging business model has profound implications for healthcare organizations and how care will be organized and delivered in the future. Pursuing value improvement requires providers to transform old operating systems and create new models of service delivery that lower costs and ensure increasingly high-quality outcomes.

To lead this transformation, healthcare executives must first confront significant operational challenges common to most health systems. These include the following:

- The rising costs of medical care resources
- The need for improved and integrated information systems

- The costs of building and sustaining ambulatory services
- The challenges of health system consolidation
- The shift from acute care hospitals
- The challenges of performance-based population health management
- The implications of increased consumer engagement and consumerism

The Continued Rise of Medical Care Resources and Costs

The rising costs of healthcare in the United States are driven largely by the ever-increasing operational expenses required to run healthcare systems. For many provider organizations, operating costs are increasing at rates that exceed revenue growth, resulting in small or negative operating margins, which are unsustainable over time.

Several operational components contribute to medical cost inflation, such as labor, supplies and capital, and facility operation.

Labor Costs

Healthcare delivery is a labor-intensive business, so providers continuously face challenges associated with

- wage inflation due to shortages in key skilled positions, including registered nurses, pharmacists, physical and occupational therapists, and numerous others;
- rising benefit expenses, particularly for employee health insurance coverage; and
- increased costs resulting from high staff turnover and recruitment expenses.

Supplies and Capital Equipment

Nonlabor expenses often represent the highest growth component of a healthcare system's operating expenses. Medical supplies represent

20 percent or more of a healthcare system's operating budget. High-growth, high-expense supply categories include the following:

- Surgical supplies associated with implants, biologics, and other devices
- Invasive cardiac supplies and devices
- Oncology drugs and other specialty pharmaceuticals
- Imaging and laboratory supplies and equipment

Facilities

Many health systems operate with outdated facilities and equipment that need renovation or replacement. The substantial investments required for these upgrades, or to service the debt associated with them, must ultimately come from philanthropy or through operating margins.

The Role of Information Systems

Information systems represent an ever-growing portion of a healthcare organization's capital investments. Significant funding is required for a wide range of applications, including the following:

- Electronic health records
- Electronic prescribing and order entry
- Clinical and operational decision support systems
- Decision support systems for population health management
- Health information exchanges
- Telemedicine

Leaders must fully leverage information technologies to streamline business processes and reduce costs. An information infrastructure is critical for healthcare systems seeking to maintain integrated and seamless processes and data flow across the enterprise. Organizations without sufficient margins will not be able to maintain the informational platform required for the future.

The Cost of Integrating Physician Services

Many healthcare systems have made substantial investments in purchasing physician practices, specialty clinics, urgent care centers, and other related ambulatory service providers. These investments are the centerpiece of a healthcare organization's drive to build integrated delivery systems that bring together hospital-based and physician office–based healthcare services. Hospital systems have many reasons for pursuing physician practice ownership, including the following:

- It provides new sources of ambulatory-based revenues.
- It preserves a hospital's primary care referral network.
- It builds physician alignment with and loyalty to the healthcare system.
- It facilitates joint business ventures between hospitals and physicians, such as comanagement agreements, bundled payment strategies, and population health management.
- It provides a foundation for cooperation in clinical and cost improvement initiatives.

Although the business case for integration is often compelling, many systems find the payback period on these investments to be much longer than originally envisioned. Healthcare systems may experience financial challenges with their physician enterprise, including

- gaps in leadership experience and competencies in managing complex, multidisciplinary physician organizations;
- lingering practice subsidies from high compensation levels and, in some cases, lower-than-planned physician productivity;

- continued leakage of patient referrals to competing organizations;
- lower-than-planned net revenues resulting from slow practice growth, payment reforms, and revenue cycle challenges;
- difficulties in consolidating practice support and administrative services; and
- challenges in blending hospital-centric cultures with physician service cultures.

The new business model will require healthcare systems to greatly improve the cost and revenue performance of their physician services enterprise and fully leverage the potential benefits of integration.

Hospital Consolidation into Large Healthcare Systems

With increasing frequency, hospital systems, through mergers and other affiliation agreements, are joining with other hospitals in their region or large national systems. Many markets today are dominated by a few large, integrated health systems.

Hospital mergers and consolidations are pursued to achieve the following goals:

- Enable joint contracting for managed care business
- Build scale and operational efficiencies
- Increase purchasing leverage for supplies and services
- Provide a broader portfolio of patient care services
- Reduce duplicative services and programs
- Expand the organization's geographic service region

Despite the many advantages of affiliation, multihospital systems are often slow to reap the full benefits. Many systems experience protracted delays in

- standardizing processes and systems to ensure consistencies in patient care services and create a unified brand;
- centralizing services beyond purchasing, patient accounts, and other support services;
- pursuing management consolidation across care sites;
- implementing clinical services consolidation to reduce duplicate programs; and
- reducing clinical practice variation across care sites and medical groups.

These delays occur most often in the early phases of system formation. During this period, individual sites and leaders frequently resist integration, preferring autonomy and retention of legacy processes and systems. Underlying these preferences are cultural norms and practices that vary across sites and are difficult to change and unify.

With increased revenue pressures, health system leaders need to focus attention on achieving the savings and revenue synergies that are possible in a multi-institutional healthcare system. For many health systems, achieving this aim requires executives to lead large-scale operational changes that are difficult to implement but necessary for the organization's future success.

The Shift from Care Delivery at Hospitals

Hospitals have long been the centerpiece of healthcare delivery. Most hospital facilities and programs have been designed primarily to support acute care services. As the most expensive component of healthcare, inpatient service utilization is a primary target for cost improvement from payers and population health initiatives. Advances in medical technologies are driving the shift of services even further from acute care to ambulatory or home care settings.

The shift from acute care has profound, long-term implications for how health systems are organized and structured, and healthcare leaders face numerous challenges as they guide organizations through this transition. For example, hospitals need to dramatically reduce inpatient bed capacity and redeploy resources to other components of the care continuum. In some cases, hospitals will eliminate acute care entirely and repurpose facilities for ambulatory care and other services.

During this transition, hospital organizations must build competencies in case management, improve inpatient throughput, and lower length-of-stay rates. Simultaneously, leaders must continuously adjust staffing and bed capacity to match reduced census levels.

Performance-Based Population Health

The shift from acute care will accelerate as the industry migrates to risk-based population health management and commensurate reimbursement. Healthcare systems must transform operations, invest in new systems and skills, and create new programs and services. The push toward population health is altering the traditional notion of margin generation for provider organizations (exhibit 1.2) and the incentives that drive provider behaviors.

Exhibit 1.2: Margin Strategies—Fee-for-Service Versus Population Health

Margin tactics driven by traditional fee-for-service:	Margin tactics driven by population health:
• Increase inpatient volume. • Increase diagnostic procedure volume. • Place priority on specialty care. • Invest capital in facilities, surgical services equipment, diagnostic tools, etc.	• Decrease inpatient volume. • Place priority on primary care. • Decrease diagnostic testing. • Invest capital in systems to monitor and "pull" patients early in disease to prevent costly and complex medical interventions.

To succeed at population health, health systems need to adopt the following approaches (Medicare.gov 2017):

- Expand clinical programs, through partnerships or acquisitions, to provide coordinated services across the full continuum of care.
- Create new medical programs designed to address the care requirements of patients with specific chronic conditions and disease states.
- Build clinically integrated networks with physicians to jointly coordinate and improve care delivery.
- Invest in information technologies, personnel, and expertise to support utilization management, health information exchanges, population analytics and predictive modeling, patient registries, and other programs.
- Implement processes and systems to support the patient-centered medical home models (AHRQ 2017).

Increased Consumerism and Consumer Engagement

Healthcare consumerism has risen in recent years out of growing public concerns and frustrations with the chronic problems plaguing the industry—rising costs, safety issues, wide variations in clinical outcomes, restricted access, and others. Consumerism continues to be fed from two primary sources: consumer-led trends and movements, and the consumer-based initiatives of government agencies, employers, health plans, and other organizations seeking to empower consumers.

In the past, a hospital's brand was formed largely on a community's subjective perceptions and the influences of physicians and advertising. Today's consumers are better informed than in the past about hospital and physician quality and cost because of the increasing availability of public performance data. The emphasis on transparency in hospital clinical and service performance measures has led to the creation of systems, such as the Medicare Hospital

Compare platform, that enable consumers to evaluate competing hospitals on the basis of multiple measures of quality, service, and cost (Medicare.gov 2017). Reported outcome data represent "brand in fact" and remove some of the subjectivity from rating hospitals. Equipped with this type of data, payers and consumers are making informed decisions in their selection of medical providers.

Increasingly, healthcare providers must institute processes, systems, and services to build engagement with medical consumers. The extent to which consumers engage in their healthcare varies, representing a progression of patient and family involvement.

Experience
Healthcare providers must enhance processes and facilities and train staff to consistently provide customer-responsive care and services. To be responsive to consumer needs, healthcare organizations need continuous feedback on programs and services through patient satisfaction surveys and focus groups. In addition to measuring satisfaction levels, healthcare systems require consumer input when planning new services, designing new facilities, or improving processes.

Engagement
Providers must engage consumers in their own care and health management. Clinicians can improve patient engagement by educating patients on their medical condition and available treatment options.

Shared Decision Making
Beyond informing patients and family members, providers should involve consumers directly in decision making related to care alternatives. Physicians and clinical staff should support efforts that engage patients in major care decisions.

Activation
Patients who are actively involved in their health management achieve better clinical outcomes than do those who receive care in a passive manner (Hibbard and Greene 2013). Effective population

health management requires informed patients who are motivated to take care of their health. Providers should inspire patients and communities to take responsibility for their health status.

IMPLICATIONS FOR PERFORMANCE IMPROVEMENT

The emerging healthcare business model reflects the new link between performance outcomes and revenues. To thrive, healthcare organizations must continuously improve in each performance dimension: cost, quality, and service. Slow, incremental improvements, while important, are not enough to transform healthcare systems to the new model. To sustain and improve operating margins, performance improvement (PI) initiatives must focus on issues that substantively reduce expenses and increase revenues. These changes must occur quickly to reposition the organization in an evolving marketplace.

The market challenges identified earlier in this chapter have substantial implications for performance improvement in a healthcare system. These implications may necessitate revisions in an organization's PI plans, priorities, and approaches. As shown in exhibit 1.3, each challenge is accompanied by specific PI issues and approaches to consider.

Health systems must reset their PI priorities and focus attention on high-impact opportunities that promise long-term benefits. While traditional operational interventions—labor productivity, revenue cycle, supply chain improvement, and so on—are still necessary, organizations increasingly need to focus attention on disruptive, high-impact changes, including

- portfolio management,
- cross-entity business process redesign,
- clinical utilization improvement,
- off-quality improvement,
- system-level consolidation, and
- growth acceleration.

Exhibit 1.3: Implications of Industry Trends for Performance Improvement Strategies

Industry Trend	Performance Improvement Implications
Costs of medical care resources continue to rise.	• Focus on process improvement and other levers that most affect labor productivity. • Institute comprehensive labor management and control systems to keep staffing levels in line with workload demand. • Optimize supply chain processes, and reduce supply variation across providers. • Continuously evaluate and drive down the costs of purchased services. • Scrutinize return on investment for large investments.
Information systems are foundational to the emerging healthcare system.	• Leverage information technologies to streamline key business processes and reduce operating expense. • Use real-time data to improve clinical and operational decision making. • Build systems to continuously monitor key performance metrics. • Employ predictive analytics to anticipate demand and risk.
Physician services integration is costly.	• Employ improvement levers that have the greatest application to ambulatory services. • Build alignment and solicit physician involvement. • Apply portfolio management principles when making investments and service line management decisions.
Hospitals are consolidating into large healthcare systems.	• Use system-level levers to achieve available cost synergies. • Focus initially on management restructuring and consolidating administrative and support functions. • Build consistencies into processes and service levels across the system. • Build an integrated culture focused on quality performance and value improvement.

(continued)

(continued from previous page)

Exhibit 1.3: Implications of Industry Trends for Performance Improvement Strategies

Industry Trend	Performance Improvement Implications
Healthcare is shifting from hospitals to external locations.	• Focus on acute care utilization improvement, including length-of-stay management and throughput. • Resize inpatient capacity to match changes in demand. • Apply portfolio management principles when making investments along the care continuum.
Performance-based population health will transform healthcare delivery.	• Institute information systems and expertise to manage medical risk. • Realign investments and operations to support an expanded care continuum. • Use portfolio management to determine make-or-buy decisions on service provision.
Consumer engagement is transforming healthcare services.	• Build systems to measure consumer satisfaction and perceptions. • Include consumer input in the design of new systems. • Focus attention on processes that most affect patient satisfaction. • Train staff on sound customer service principles. • Engage consumers in their own healthcare.

These initiatives often bring high levels of change to healthcare systems and can be challenging for some leaders, physicians, and staff. This work requires new resources, expertise, and management systems support. For some organizations, these changes require a new leadership framework and PI approach.

CHAPTER 2

Assessing the Starting Point

SOME HEALTH SYSTEMS are better than others at managing large-scale performance improvement (PI) projects and achieving targeted results. Myriad factors, both internal and external, account for the success or failure of PI projects. While progressive health systems share a number of common disciplines and capabilities, five core competencies bear the most significant impact on PI achievement:

- Performance improvement leadership
- Workforce engagement
- Consumer engagement
- Physician engagement
- Data-driven management

Effective transformation begins with an honest assessment of an organization's strengths and weaknesses in these areas.

PERFORMANCE IMPROVEMENT LEADERSHIP

Organizational competencies emanate from, and are most influenced by, the collective capabilities of the leadership team. High-performing healthcare organizations build leadership teams with the skills and personal attributes required to set strategic vision and direction and execute tactical initiatives to achieve organizational goals. Effective management teams foster a corporate ethos of continuous performance improvement and inspire others in the organization to lead.

Executives can take several actions to ensure the success of a PI initiative, including the following:

- *Build a shared PI philosophy and approach.* Leaders should adopt, communicate, and adhere to a unifying framework and approach to performance improvement. Models such as Lean, Plan-Do-Check-Act, and Six Sigma provide organizations with proven processes, useful tools, and a uniting philosophy to guide leaders and focus the organization.
- *Lead by example.* Progressive leaders consistently demonstrate knowledge of and commitment to PI by promoting and participating in continuous improvement work. Key leadership decisions are consistent with the espoused philosophy and culture of continuous improvement.
- *Build a culture of accountability.* Effective leaders consistently hold themselves and their leadership team accountable for performance. Organizations should build a culture of accountability characterized by clearly understood performance goals at every level. Accountability is sustained by
  - setting tactical targets and goals and assigning responsibilities and deadlines,
  - incentivizing leaders to perform as measured by relevant goals,
  - building disciplines around budget development and compliance, and

- practicing data-driven decision making and requiring the same of others.
- *Invest in people.* Successful PI is driven by leaders and staff equipped with the right knowledge, skills, and tools to achieve specified goals. Organizations should invest in training leaders and staff on the improvement model and how tools and principles are applied to improve healthcare operations and outcomes. Managers should have the support of internal consultants with deep technical expertise to assist with staff development and facilitate improvement projects. Internal consultants should have specialized skills in analytics, PI tools, and PI methodologies that can be taught to other staff and appropriately applied to performance issues.
- *Focus on high-performing practices.* Successful leaders continuously seek knowledge of high-performing practices in the industry and lead the adoption of these practices. Organizations should focus on identifying internal and external practices and systems that can be adopted systematically. Benchmarking should include the use of comparative industry data, surveys, and shared practices with peer organizations.
- *Build a PI strategy and plan.* Performance improvement should support and align with the strategic goals and initiatives of the organization. In this regard, health systems should formulate annual PI strategies and goals as part of the organization's planning process. A performance improvement plan should define a portfolio of PI projects encapsulating all business units of the enterprise. The plan should identify improvement goals supported by clearly defined metrics and numeric targets. Additionally, the PI plan should delineate how PI resources and support will be apportioned to support the improvement initiatives.

WORKFORCE ENGAGEMENT

Effective healthcare service delivery can only occur through a protean workforce that is satisfied and motivated. High-performing healthcare executives continuously sustain and strengthen workforce engagement. Specifically, these leaders

- build a transparent and supportive work culture that fosters collaboration and diversity;
- continuously communicate to all levels of the organization, particularly during major PI initiatives;
- solicit staff feedback and involvement in PI initiatives and provide forums for employees to voice concerns and ideas;
- commit resources to associates' development and job growth;
- consistently provide feedback on performance and follow through on promises; and
- institute effective systems to recognize and reward individual and group performance.

Maintaining workforce engagement can be challenging during a major PI initiative. These efforts may be seen as threatening to middle managers and line staff, as such initiatives can result in staff reductions, redesigned roles, changes in managerial responsibilities, or redeployment of staff to other departments or sites.

When an organization undertakes a major PI initiative, executives must recognize that middle managers and staff will have varying perceptions, ideas, and concerns about the project. As shown in exhibit 2.1, at the outset of a PI initiative, individuals typically fall into one of four groups along the engagement continuum: defiant, skeptical, tractable, and empowered.

Defiant staff, representing a small portion of the affected workforce, act in an uncooperative, openly negative manner and seek to undermine the organization's improvement goals. Frequently,

Exhibit 2.1: Measuring Workforce Engagement

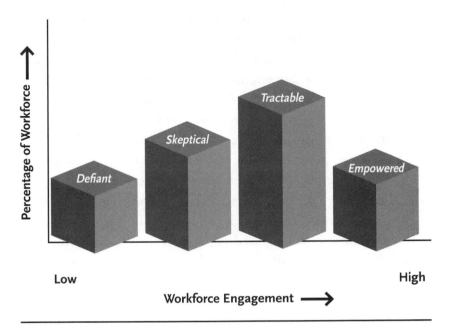

defiant individuals are connected to the upper stratum of the organization's social network and influence others' perceptions and opinions. When possible, leaders should preemptively engage these individuals to understand the basis for their dissatisfaction. In some cases, defiant staff may have insights that are useful to the initiative; their contrarian view may reveal leadership blind spots or help the organization avoid unseen mistakes down the road.

Other defiant individuals may simply demonstrate a lack of willingness to cooperate. Some defiant staff may be in positions of authority and thus pose barriers for improvement. In these cases, both the organization and the individual may best be served by parting ways.

Typically representing a higher percentage of staff than the defiant group, the *skeptics* need to be encouraged to bring them along to the point of committing willingly to PI. Communication regarding the "why" of the initiative must occur early in the process for this group. The organization needs to understand the basis for the skepticism and proactively address each valid issue raised. Skeptics can be useful as members of collaborative teams in providing alternative points of view. Skepticism is often based on the experiences and shortcomings of previous PI initiatives, so skeptics need to be convinced that the new initiative is different from previous efforts and that the organization will act to prevent past errors.

The *tractable* group typically represents the largest component of the workforce. This group harbors some degree of skepticism but has an open mind for change. Like other groups, tractable staff need to understand the reasons for performance improvement, what goals and outcomes are anticipated, and the process for achieving them. Tractable staff and managers have knowledge of processes and systems and can serve as effective collaborative team members and leaders.

A portion of leaders and staff will embrace change from the outset. This *empowered* group, which recognizes the need for new or reconceived processes, may include those leaders who have been pressing the organization to change. A small number of this group may exhibit enthusiasm for change but are not fully engaged. When possible, empowered staff should be assigned to leadership and collaborative team roles. Especially important is that top leaders demonstrate enthusiasm for the change, spearhead organizational communication efforts, and convert the detractors into tractable and empowered staff.

Over the life of a project, leaders should build and maintain consensus and buy-in across the organization. Ultimately, people want to understand how future changes will affect them and their role in the organization. Before launching a major PI initiative, leaders should assess workforce engagement to determine if any job categories, departments, or business units are resistant to the PI process and goals. Surveys and focus groups can provide important insights into satisfaction and perceptions, informing

PI leaders about barriers to overcome, available champions to drive engagement, messages to communicate, and cohort groups to address.

CONSUMER ENGAGEMENT

High-performing healthcare systems are effective at engaging patients and families in their medical care and in improving processes and systems that support care. These organizations consistently earn high patient satisfaction levels and maintain strong brand recognition in the communities they serve.

Specifically, high-performing organizations are adept at

- listening to the voice of the customer (or VOC, as used in Six Sigma terminology) by consistently monitoring community perception and patient satisfaction through multimodal methods;
- understanding distinct market segments and patient populations served, and designing programs and services around the specific needs of these groups;
- using consumer information to identify and improve process and service gaps;
- soliciting community member feedback and input routinely when planning new services or improving existing programs;
- focusing on building consumer engagement and shared decision making in patients' care to improve quality outcomes;
- investing in programs and outreach services to build awareness of and loyalty to the communities served;
- investing in service training and scripting for associates who interface with patients and families; and
- instituting service recovery procedures for follow-up on adverse service events.

Performance improvement initiatives should produce responsive processes and systems that meet the requirements and expectations of the patients served better than the organization has done in the past. Before launching a PI initiative, those leading the effort must understand the degree to which the organization is currently meeting these requirements. Consumer information gathered toward this end helps

- reveal problem areas and process issues that impact patient service;
- identify key customer requirements for teams that are focused on process improvement;
- inform collaborative teams focused on growth or service improvement initiatives; and
- improve medical compliance, lower readmissions, and reduce the frequency of off-quality events.

Off-quality events are any occurrences of unfavorable clinical or service outcomes. Off-quality improvement is lever 12, covered extensively in chapter 8.

PHYSICIAN ENGAGEMENT

Healthcare systems cannot succeed without building alignment with their affiliated medical staff. The importance of physicians to healthcare systems is self-evident:

- Physicians have primary control over the medical care provided by a healthcare system and thereby drive most of the operating expenses.
- Surgery and other specialist-based services generate most of the contribution margin for healthcare systems.

- Primary care physicians are instrumental in driving referrals to specialists and hospital inpatient and outpatient services.
- Affiliated physicians have a significant impact on the brand and quality (real and perceived) of a healthcare organization.

High-performing healthcare systems recognize that performance initiatives affect the physicians and practices with which they align. Involvement of medical leaders and affiliated clinical staff is recommended to foster buy-in for strategic initiative and operational changes. Like system associates, the medical staff have their share of skeptics and detractors when a PI initiative is launched. At the start of a major PI initiative, an important first step is to evaluate the degree of alignment that exists between the organization and its physicians.

As shown in exhibit 2.2, physician alignment with a health system ranges from informal relationships to integrated partnerships with shared goals and risks. Successfully aligned relationships are those supported by data and information that help clarify market opportunities and set strategic priorities. Additionally, organizations need to gather data on physician performance on an ongoing basis, in part to identify medical staff members to pursure for greater alignment. These physicians should be high-quality clinicians who have influence with other physicians and are supportive of a health system's mission and goals.

To assess how the organization's present state of physician alignment affects its performance, seek to answer the following questions:

- Do physicians tend to support organizational performance initiatives, or do they actively resist such changes?
- Are hospital-based physicians (e.g., pathologists, radiologists, intensivists, hospitalists, emergency

Exhibit 2.2: Dimensions of Physician Alignment

	Filter and Find	Work with Prioritized Physicians	Work with Tested and Trusted Physicians
	• Tools used to identify highest-value physicians • Tools used to find physicians with the most influence in the practicing community • Structured interactions • Maximized time and resources devoted to physician alignment	• Improved scores on publicly reported hospital measures • Targeted patient safety initiatives • Targeted growth strategies • Targeted utilization strategies • Select supply chain initiatives • Targeted referral strategies	• Integrated strategic/growth plans • Integrated financial success plans • Integrated quality plans • Integrated safety plans • Joint ventures • Most effective resource allocation
	• Friendly, social • Priorities based on intuition • Priorities based on "noise"	• Collaborations developed, but may not leverage resources or time spent with physicians	• Financial plans that may have a win–lose solution • Growth plans that may have a win–lose solution • Defensive joint ventures
	Relationship	Collaboration	Integration
	Tactical		Strategic

Highest Value
Highest Alignment

Fact Based

Increasing Alignment →

Increasing Alignment →

Intuition Based

Lowest Value
Lowest Alignment

department physicians) engaged in productivity and performance improvement in their areas of responsibility?

- Are physicians supportive of and involved in initiatives to improve patient access and throughput in their practices and in the hospital?
- Are the incentive plans of the employed physicians based, at least in part, on individual and practice productivity and quality goals?
- Are surgeons and anesthesiologists engaged in and aligned with PI initiatives for surgical procedures and supportive of efforts to improve operating room and staff utilization, room turnover, and block scheduling utilization?
- Do physician executives, including the chief medical officer, provide the leadership required for PI and organizational transformation?
- Does the organization have current data and systems in place to measure physician satisfaction and perceptions?
- Are transparent mechanisms in place with which to communicate with the medical staff?

Physician leaders should be tapped to guide or support PI initiatives. Those who fill these roles should be in positions of authority and have the respect of the medical staff. Physician leaders help the organization by

- providing direction and leadership for PI initiatives, particularly in areas related to clinical quality and patient care;
- participating in and leading collaborative teams, particularly teams focused on clinical utilization, patient throughput, and length-of-stay rate improvement;
- facilitating communications with the medical staff; and
- interfacing with other physicians on clinical issues such as changes in preference supply items, formulary

changes, clinical pathway development, and other patient management issues.

DATA-DRIVEN MANAGEMENT

To be effective, the management of PI initiatives must include the accurate and consistent measurement of performance throughout the organization. High-performing healthcare systems are adept at using data and information to inform decision making and measure ongoing organizational performance. Leaders must maintain effective measurement systems to

- accurately measure and report clinical quality outcomes,
- track labor and other operational expenses,
- capture workload counts across diverse service areas and accurately project future workload volumes,
- use standard data platforms as a basis for internal and external benchmarking,
- measure profit and loss performance for each component of the service portfolio,
- monitor actual performance against budget and quantify variances,
- measure staff and physician satisfaction and engagement, and
- measure patient satisfaction and perceptions.

Effective organizations use a comprehensive, balanced set of performance metrics that accurately measure key dimensions of performance. They typically employ a layered set of key performance indicators (KPIs) that track performance for the entire organization as well as its divisions, service lines, departments, programs, and cross-functional processes. Most metrics are monitored by a process for measuring planned versus actual performance. KPI information should include trended data and provide comparisons against historical performance.

Healthcare organizations must maintain data transparency and accessibility for decision makers to make timely, informed decisions. Up-to-date performance data should be continuously shared with key stakeholders, including leadership, staff, and physicians.

Organizational leaders should have a high degree of competency in performance measurement, including developing metrics and understanding, analyzing, and interpreting performance data for their areas of responsibility. They should be assisted by competent analytical staff and efficient systems to support data mining and knowledge management.

Organizations should also have decision support systems in place to predict future performance and facilitate preemptive action, such as changes in strategy and tactics, contingency planning, and the automatic triggering of predefined response plans.

Data and performance metrics are a critical component of PI initiatives. Performance data and information are needed to

- identify and measure performance gaps to guide improvement teams and initiatives,
- seize economic gains from opportunities identified through PI initiatives, and
- track actual performance gains after implementation.

PRELAUNCH ORGANIZATIONAL ASSESSMENT

The strength of an organization's core competencies can largely determine the success of performance improvement projects. If gaps exist in one or more competency, implementing PI system and process changes is difficult. Leaders must preemptively confront these issues and build proficiencies concurrent with the PI initiative.

Health system leaders should gauge the organization's current performance levels against the five core competencies—PI leadership, workforce engagement, consumer engagement, physician engagement, and data-driven management—before launching a major PI effort. This assessment provides a means for gaining shared understanding of performance gaps and focuses attention on areas that need to be addressed. Appendix A provides a sample assessment tool to identify areas of competency strengths and gaps. The survey should be completed by senior leaders and discussed as a group. From this exercise, the team can draw conclusions on areas requiring attention during the redesign and implementation phases.

A prelaunch assessment should also include a quantitative review of the organization's current operating and market performance. Such a review may include a summary of the following PI elements:

- Current versus planned profitability and operating margins for the organization as a whole and for key operating units
- Operating cost trends and performance against budget
- Current engagement and satisfaction scores for key constituent groups, including patients, staff, and physicians
- Overall clinical quality metrics, such as the Centers for Medicare & Medicaid Services (CMS 2017b) Quality Core Measures
- An assessment of competitors and market share data for key services

Prelaunch assessments may also include performance benchmarking analyses. Most healthcare organizations use comparative data to evaluate performance in many areas of the operation, including labor, supplies, clinical utilization, patient satisfaction, and financial and clinical quality performance. Benchmark data are used by organizations and leaders to

- understand how performance compares to peer hospitals,
- gauge performance gaps relative to competitors,
- set performance standards and budgets,

- identify cost and PI opportunities, and
- identify high-performing industry practices.

In addition to external comparisons, the organization may benchmark the current state to historical performance or, in the case of large systems, compare the internal performance of similar programs or departments.

The organizational assessment is a crucial first step in the performance improvement process. Assessing the current state at the start of a PI effort provides insights into opportunities and targets, competency gaps that must be addressed, and strengths that need to be leveraged. A summary of the assessment should be reviewed by the senior leadership team to ensure that its members understand the need for change, agree with the targets and areas to pursue, and buy into the redesign process.

The assessment also provides leaders the information needed to communicate

- business and market conditions, or the organization's current financial position, that require the organization to improve operational performance;
- improvement opportunities that have been identified and the data and rationale for how these conclusions were reached;
- the process whereby improvement opportunities will be pursued and the timing requirements for the project; and
- roles and responsibilities of leadership going forward.

IDENTIFICATION OF IMPROVEMENT OPPORTUNITIES AND GOAL SETTING

In the initial phase of a major performance improvement project, an organization should identify operational gaps and quantify the magnitude of the improvement opportunity. Performance gaps are typically expressed as financial opportunity—cost savings or revenue growth—but can also represent incremental gains in clinical or service quality measures, cycle time improvement, and other metrics.

Performance improvement initiatives should focus on areas that will yield the greatest benefit to patients and the organization. For example, leaders can identify departmental productivity issues and improvement opportunities from multiple sources, including the following:

- *Benchmarking.* The department or program performs below similar benchmark institutions relative to cost or quality outcomes.
- *Productivity monitoring.* The department's productivity has been trending downward over the past several reporting periods.
- *Budget.* The department consistently exceeds its operating budget.
- *Workload.* Workload volumes have dropped without a corresponding reduction in staffing and operating expenses.
- *Premium labor.* The department uses a high number of overtime hours or uses a high portion of agency or contract hours.
- *Access and throughput.* The department has process issues with patient access and throughput that drive up staffing costs.
- *Opportunity size.* Opportunities should be prioritized in part on the basis of the size of the potential economic or quality gain. Large departments with high-paid professional staff generally have more savings potential than support areas and small departments have.

Leadership should also consider additional factors when targeting areas for improvement. Low patient or physician satisfaction could be an artifact of poor processes, insufficient training, or any of a number of other factors. For example, employee dissatisfaction and turnover could indicate problems with staffing, role design, or leadership, which also results in reduced productivity.

Categories of Performance Improvement Opportunities

Performance improvement opportunities in a health system can be grouped into seven categories:

- *Labor expense*—lowering hours and labor costs per unit of service, reducing premium pay use
- *Nonlabor expense*—lowering costs of supplies, purchased services, and professional fees
- *Clinical utilization improvement*—reducing cost per case and length of stay
- *Off-quality improvement*—reducing costs and incidence of off-quality events
- *Portfolio management*—strengthening the performance and mix of services provided
- *Revenue cycle improvement*—maximizing net revenues through improving components of the revenue cycle
- *Revenue growth*—increasing top-line revenues through growth in market share and patient volumes

The prelaunch assessment should include an estimate of the opportunity and an improvement target. The format for summarizing this information can vary, depending on the scope of the improvement project and how the organization chooses to structure the initiative. Exhibit 2.3 is an example of target setting for a hospital system. This organization identified seven potential initiatives, three of which focus on major service lines. Each initiative includes a measure of the total expense base reflecting the scope of areas under evaluation. The projected savings percentages are

Exhibit 2.3: Example of Improvement Target Setting

Potential Initiatives	Expense Base	Improvement		Projected Savings		Projected Added CM*	
		Low	High	Low	High	Low	High
Portfolio review	$14,379,930	2.8%	6.3%	$402,638	$905,936	$321,198	$392,562
Cardiac service line	$20,014,145	3.0%	6.3%	$600,424	$1,260,891	$427,464	$769,435
Neurosciences service line	$9,822,419	2.4%	4.6%	$235,738	$451,831	$42,830	$77,094
Orthopedics service line	$9,216,980	4.4%	9.0%	$405,547	$829,528	$54,650	$109,300
Revenue cycle	$6,105,014	2.0%	4.5%	$122,100	$274,726	$3,200,000	$6,200,000
Supplies	$24,679,089	9.2%	17.4%	$2,270,476	$4,294,161	$0	$0
Productivity	$19,882,380	7.9%	15.7%	$1,570,708	$3,121,534	$0	$0
Overall	**$104,099,957**	**5.4%**	**10.7%**	**$5,607,632**	**$11,138,607**	**$4,046,142**	**$7,548,391**

* Calculated on the basis of additional cases through improved length of stay or growth through portfolio enhancement; does not include increased case management (CM) from cost reductions.

based on a combination of internal performance targets and external benchmarking results. Calculating the target as a range is useful to identify both the minimum improvement required and a stretch target. This example also includes a potential added contribution margin that is targeted on the basis of improvements in the revenue cycle and growth opportunities. The leadership team can use these targets to charter collaborative teams for each of the seven PI initiative categories.

The endpoint of the assessment phase is achieving consensus among the executive leadership team on the findings and conclusions. Specifically, agreement should be reached on the following points:

- The internal and external factors driving the need for margin improvement
- The organization's identified core strengths and gaps
- The conclusions from the quantitative assessment, including support for external benchmarks
- The specific PI initiatives to be embarked on and the recommended targets for each
- Timelines, including start and end dates

CHAPTER 3

A New Framework for Healthcare Performance Improvement

HEALTHCARE PERFORMANCE IMPROVEMENT (PI) has evolved over the past three decades in both theory and practice. During this time, the industry has adopted and discarded different improvement processes and frameworks on the basis of new thinking and approaches that have proved sucessful in other industries.

Exhibit 3.1 is a partial listing of improvement models and principles that have been prominent in healthcare over the past 30 years. Each of these approaches has specific key principles and methodologies that are complementary to or overlap with other approaches.

Most healthcare organizations adopt improvement models to serve as a unifying philosophy and approach to PI. Today, Lean methods are used in a majority of hospitals and health systems. Many Lean principles build on the foundational work of Deming (1986), Juran (1989), Crosby (1986), and other thought leaders of the total quality management movement. Six Sigma's DMAIC (define, measure, analyze, improve, and control) framework is another approach that is frequently used with Lean initiatives (Wedgwood 2007; Dean 2013; Chalice 2007).

Important lessons can be gleaned from ideas and approaches that were used in the past. For example, reengineering was a dominant approach to PI in the mid-1990s (Hammer 1990). Although reengineering terminology has long fallen out of fashion, the lessons of

Exhibit 3.1: Performance Improvement Methods and Tools in Healthcare Services

Performance Improvement Models and Methods	Time Period	Key Principles
Management engineering (Smalley 1982; Larson 2014)	Late 1970s–1990s	• Scientific management method • Productivity management and monitoring • Work measurement and engineered work standards • Activity-based cost accounting
Total quality management (Deming 1986; Juran 1989; Crosby 1986)	Late 1980s–1990s	• Focus on quality/ quality is free • Focus on customer requirements • Culture of involvement/ drive out fear
Plan-Do-Check-Act (Deming 1986; Leebov and Ersoz 2003)	1980s–present	• Continuous improvement • Performance measurement and checking of results
Baldrige National Quality Program (NIST 2017)	1980s–present	• Achieving optimal results through successful leadership, strategy, operations, workforce, and customer focus integration and execution

(continued)

(continued from previous page)

Exhibit 3.1: Performance Improvement Methods and Tools in Healthcare Services

Performance Improvement Models and Methods	Time Period	Key Principles
Reengineering (Hammer 1990)	1990s–early 2000s	• Challenging fundamental assumptions about how work should be organized and delivered • Radically redesigning business processes to achieve substantial improvements in performance
Patient-focused care (Lathrop 1993; Leander 1996)	Late 1980s–mid-1990s	• Service redeployment • Job design and multiskilled workforce • Service reaggregation
Performance benchmarking (Reider 2000)	Late 1980s–present	• Comparative benchmarking • Identification of best practices • Internal benchmarking
Six Sigma (DMAIC in particular) and Lean (Wedgwood 2007; Dean 2013; Chalice 2007)	Late 1980s–present	• Reduce variation • Reduce waste • Statistical process control

Note: DMAIC = define, measure, analyze, improve, and control.

radical redesign and challenging assumptions about work performance remain valid in today's healthcare environment. Similarly, the patient-focused care principles of service redeployment, service reaggregation, and multiskilling are applicable to hospital and health system improvement today (Lathrop 1993; Leander 1996).

The framework presented in this book is inspired, in part, by concepts and approaches from the past that are still relevant. The improvement levers and collaborative team approach are not intended to be an alternative to well-established improvement models. Rather, they are specific interventions and methods that can fit in an organization's established improvement framework. These levers represent ways to accelerate the existing improvement process by focusing leaders on the key issues relevant to all healthcare systems. The framework reduces the time required to identify problems and prioritize opportunities.

Regardless of which improvement approach is adopted, organizations need a framework that, at a minimum, defines the following:

- The key tenets and rationale for continuous quality and performance improvement and its criticality to the organization's mission and success.
- The sequential phases and steps in the improvement process, from initial assessment through implementation, that should be followed by leaders and PI teams.
- The roles and uses of data measurement as a requirement for assessing opportunity, measuring progress, and tracking ongoing performance.
- The importance of service excellence and the need to design processes and systems to meet external customer requirements. For healthcare organizations, this includes a focus on processes and systems that affect
  - patients,
  - physicians,
  - payer groups,
  - regulators, and
  - other provider partners.

- The roles and responsibilities of internal stakeholder groups in the improvement process. Health system stakeholder groups include the
  - board of directors,
  - executive leadership,
  - middle managers,
  - line staff,
  - physicians, and
  - suppliers.
- The principles and protocols used to identify, assign, and lead PI initiatives.
- The aspirational cultural values of an organization (e.g., transparency, involvement, empowerment).

ISSUES IN HEALTH SYSTEM PERFORMANCE IMPROVEMENT

Although many healthcare organizations adopt a PI philosophy, the results they obtain can vary considerably. Performance improvement initiatives can tie up time and resources, sometimes without producing tangible results. Some underlying issues that impede healthcare PI include the following:

- *Focus on structure and process rather than on results.* Most healthcare leaders are adept at adopting new management ideas and approaches. They embrace the philosophy, language, and process, and they support training for managers and associates. These efforts often generate considerable activity but yield subpar performance gains.
- *Lack of prioritization.* Many organizations fail to prioritize opportunities that yield the greatest benefit to the organization and patients served. Frequently, leaders focus on small, easy-to-implement ideas while avoiding challenging opportunities with greater performance impact.

- *Lack of engagement.* Large-scale improvement requires the buy-in and involvement of a health system's key constituent groups. These include the management team, associates, physicians, and the board, among others. PI projects typically fail if these groups do not support the project or are not actively engaged in the process.
- *Lack of urgency.* Healthcare systems are slow to move and usually do not undertake large-scale improvement without a degree of financial or strategic urgency. Leaders must create urgency by communicating the reasons driving the need for change and by setting deadlines and targets for managers and improvement teams to meet.
- *Lack of measurement.* Performance improvement requires disciplined measurement and monitoring. Organizations that do not measure performance cannot know if performance is improving, getting worse, or staying the same.
- *Lack of accountability.* A fundamental aspect of successful PI efforts is senior leadership securing buy-in from managers and holding them accountable for their results. Executives must also hold themselves accountable for meeting goals and should institute processes for regularly reviewing performance metrics. Many organizations tie leader compensation, in part, to achieving PI goals.

To succeed in today's healthcare environment, providers need PI processes and strategies that overcome these issues.

A NEW PERFORMANCE IMPROVEMENT FRAMEWORK

Programs and services in a health system are highly interconnected with, and dependent on, other organizational functions and operations. Health services delivery requires continuous orchestration and coordinated flow of patients, staff, equipment, supplies, and information across numerous departments, services, and care sites.

A leader's ability to manage performance in his department depends, in part, on the effective workflow of and support from other departments. An emergency department (ED) director, for example, has control over the staffing and workflow in the ED. Her ability to optimize ED staff productivity and patient throughput, however, is hampered if the systems for expediting emergency admissions to the nursing units are ineffective.

This example illustrates how PI opportunities can arise at different levels and with varying scope in the organization. Coffey (2005) suggests that five levels are typical in a healthcare system: patient, department or unit, hospital, multi-institutional/multiorganizational system, and virtually integrated health system. The focus of this book is on PI that takes place at three similar levels: the department or program (process) level, the cross-functional or cross-site (structure) level, and the cross-market or cross-population (portfolio) level (see exhibit 3.2).

Process changes include the routine operational modifications leaders make daily in their specific areas of responsibilities. Regarding productivity, process initiatives represent department-level changes in work schedules, role design, and workflow improvements that improve staff utilization and service to patients. The organizational impact from process-level changes depends on the size and complexity of the department. Organizations in the early stages of PI should first focus on building department-level processes and systems. For health systems, this means prioritizing improvements that

- streamline key processes in a department or program,
- strengthen departmental supply and inventory management systems,
- reconfigure department work areas to improve workflow and capacity,
- redesign roles to meet changes in work requirements, and
- improve labor productivity through improved personnel scheduling and role design.

Exhibit 3.2: Three Levels of Health System Performance Improvement

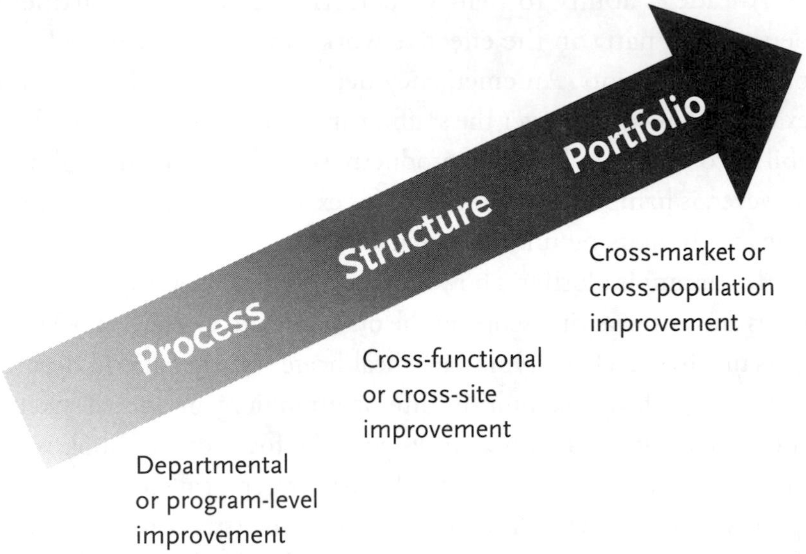

Process — Departmental or program-level improvement

Structure — Cross-functional or cross-site improvement

Portfolio — Cross-market or cross-population improvement

At some point, health system leaders may find that further improvement can only occur by addressing processes and systems that cross over into other areas of the organization. These improvement opportunities occur at the second, or *structure*, level. Change levers (discussed at length in the next section) that drive structural improvement represent operational interventions that are executed among functions both in a facility and across multiple facilities of a health system.

As hospitals, physician groups, and post-acute organizations merge to create large, complex, integrated systems, operational improvements derive increasingly from structure-level changes. These interventions are categorized as structural because they often challenge and alter the foundational assumptions of hospital and health system processes and organization. Multientity health systems form, in large part, to achieve the scale and efficiencies that are unachievable for independent facilities.

Structural improvement levers address the following essential areas:

- Leveraging the advantages of system scale to rationalize staffing and other resources across multiple entities
- Improving key business processes to enhance service continuity across functions and system entities
- Improving case cost performance and contribution margin by reducing unnecessary utilization of clinical services
- Improving quality outcomes and minimizing the occurrence of off-quality events
- Building effective processes and systems for managing enterprisewide supplies and other nonlabor expenses

Structural improvement projects are often complex, requiring a great deal of time and effort and the involvement of large, diverse groups of leaders and staff. When executed effectively, structural improvement initiatives can yield substantial gains in organizational performance.

Beyond process and structural changes, further PI is achieved through alterations in the portfolio of services and programs provided by a health system. *Portfolio*-level changes occur when health systems reconfigure and redesign programs and services to respond to changes in market demand.

The aim of portfolio management is to maintain a service offering that meets market demand and maximizes revenues and margins. For a healthcare system, portfolio improvement levers are used to

- inform decisions on which services to expand, contract, or divest;
- determine which components of the care continuum should be produced internally versus by a partnering entity;
- identify strategic marketing opportunities and tactical growth initiatives to build top-line revenues; and

- improve net revenues and margins through enhancements to the organization's revenue cycle.

Portfolio improvement is a growing area of focus for large healthcare systems. As accountable care and population health initiatives transform healthcare delivery, health systems must institute changes to their service portfolio by reducing investments in existing programs and building new programs and capabilities. Similarly, growth and revenue cycle improvements are necessary for building and sustaining operating margins.

CHANGE LEVERS

Change levers are specific interventions employed at different levels of the organization. As shown in exhibit 3.3, 18 PI levers can be applied to healthcare operations. A detailed description of each lever is provided in appendix B. While depicted as discreet strategies, change levers are often employed with other levers. For example, process improvement frequently drives changes in role design, improvements in facility layout, and efforts to match resources to work demand.

The 18 levers are divided into two categories: supply and demand. Many of the levers deal with balancing the *supply* of labor and resources for a given demand. These interventions are employed to effectively match the right resources to the right demand at the right time. From a portfolio perspective, supply levers can also identify services that should be provided by an outside entity and those that should be eliminated.

Healthcare leaders also seek operational improvement by influencing the *demand* for the work. Demand levers are used to redistribute workload to reduce variation and improve service, reduce demand to minimize non-value-added work, and grow demand to improve resource utilization and contribution margins.

Exhibit 3.3: 18 Performance Improvement Levers for Healthcare Organizations

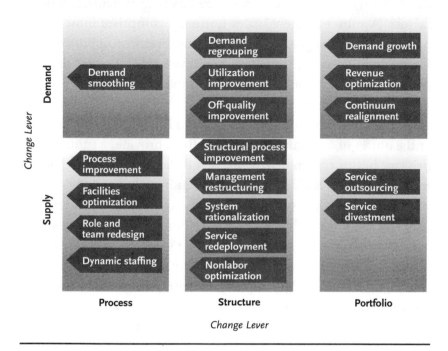

PERFORMANCE LEVERS AND HEALTH SYSTEM FUNCTIONS

Most hospitals, physician offices, and other medical services are similar with respect to structure, processes, and operational issues. Most hospitals, for example, confront similar operational challenges related to

- scheduling and throughput in surgical services,
- patient throughput and staffing in emergency services,
- patient discharge processes and room turnover, and
- staffing and scheduling for acute care units.

For every functional area in a health system, several operational issues are predictable and common to most organizations. The impact of these issues varies with the size and complexity of the department, the demand dynamics, location and facility requirements, and other factors. A subset of these issues normally comprises most of the operational challenges and resulting improvement opportunities. Consequently, specific improvement levers offer the best or most effective approach for addressing improvement needs in a given department or function.

The primary operational improvement levers can be determined at the outset of a PI initiative. Appendix C provides a summary of primary health system departments and the change levers that are most effective for achieving improvement in each. Focusing on this subset can minimize assessment time and quickly point leaders and teams to solutions with the highest likelihood of improvement success. For example, a physician practice improvement team should initially concentrate on the seven areas highlighted in exhibit 3.4—those that most closely pertain to ambulatory services. Each lever is paired with a corresponding primary question to address. The team can use these questions to brainstorm and identify areas of focus and redesign alternatives.

SYSTEM-LEVEL GAP CLOSURE PLAN

Performance improvement strategies must address an increasingly broad range of operational issues and extend over multiple years. Exhibit 3.5 is an example of a four-year financial gap closure strategy for a regional healthcare system. The chief financial officer of this organization prepared a forecast of the organization's expected decline in operating margins under a scenario in which net revenues per inpatient case for all payers would approach prevailing Medicare rates. On the basis of this scenario, the organization's operating margins would drop by $35 million in the first year and grow to $68 million by the fourth year.

Exhibit 3.4: Key Improvement Levers—Physician Enterprise Example

Improvement Lever	Key Questions	Brainstorming Ideas
Process improvement	What can we change in our processes to improve patient throughput in our clinics?	Improve check-in process, collect data previsit, perform waiting room rounding.
Role design	How can we redesign roles among our clinical and nonclinical staff to increase staffing flexibility and utilization?	Cross-train medical assistant (MA) role with the front-desk role; have MA perform patient data collection.
Dynamic staffing	What staffing models give us the most cost-effective team design and meet the needs of our patients?	Increase use of physician extender staffing.
Demand smoothing	How can we schedule patients in a manner that balances workload with staff schedules while ensuring access for our patients?	Standardize office hours and scheduling protocols for physicians, and introduce central scheduling to balance demand across practices.
System rationalization	What clinic-based administrative functions can be offered more effectively as a centralized service?	Consolidate administrative functions (e.g., medical records management, authorizations management, coding).
Divestment	What underperforming clinics need to be reduced or eliminated as a result of changing market demand?	Target 2–3 underperforming practices for shutdown or reduction in scale.
Demand growth	What can we do to increase access to accommodate unmet demand in our clinics?	Open new practice in western suburbs.

Exhibit 3.5: Example of a System-Level Gap Closure Plan

Performance Improvement Initiative	Improvement Levers	Economic Improvement Targets				Notes
		Year 1	Year 2	Year 3	Year 4	
Labor productivity	1–Process improvement, 2–Structural process improvement, 3–Facilities optimization, 4–Demand smoothing, 5–Demand regrouping, 6–Role and team redesign, 7–Dynamic staffing, 10–Service redeployment	$10,450,000	$11,495,000	$12,644,500	$13,908,000	Target 35th percentile benchmark staffing in all departments.
Leadership restructuring and functional consolidation	8–Management restructuring, 9–System rationalization, 10–Service redeployment	$2,000,000	$5,340,000	$9,450,000	$10,395,000	Start with regional management restructuring.
Supplies and purchased services	11–Nonlabor optimization	$3,500,000	$4,025,000	$4,628,500	$5,323,000	Examples include physician preference, commodities, pharmaceuticals, purchased services.
Portfolio review	16–Service outsourcing, 17–Service divestment, 18–Continuum realignment	$500,000	$1,000,000	$3,200,000	$4,000,000	Will take longer to implement.
Clinical utilization	13–Utilization improvement	$2,500,000	$3,250,000	$4,387,500	$6,142,000	Focus on LOS for Medicare patients and cost per case in cardiac, neurosciences, and orthopedic service lines.
Quality improvement	12–Off-quality improvement	$0	$1,950,000	$2,340,000	$2,808,000	Focus on reducing readmissions, DVT, VAP.
Revenue cycle	15–Revenue optimization	$5,800,000	$5,280,000	$5,280,000	$5,280,000	Improve charge capture and coding; reduce denials.
Growth	14–Demand growth	$2,580,000	$2,760,500	$2,953,000	$3,614,000	Reduce patient leakage; build service line referrals.

Hospital- and System-Led Initiatives

(continued)

(*continued from previous page*)

Exhibit 3.5: Example of a System-Level Gap Closure Plan

Physician Enterprise Initiatives

Performance Improvement Initiative	Improvement Levers	Economic Improvement Targets				Notes
		Year 1	Year 2	Year 3	Year 4	
Labor productivity	1–Process improvement, 2–Structural process improvement, 3–Facilities optimization, 4–Demand smoothing, 5–Demand regrouping, 6–Role and team redesign, 7–Dynamic staffing, 10–Service redeployment, 17–Service divestment	$1,580,000	$1,896,000	$2,370,000	$2,844,000	Improve staffing to 65th percentile against MGMA benchmarks; divest low-performing practices; consolidate support and administrative services.
Revenue cycle	2–Structural process improvement, 15–Revenue optimization	$1,500,000	$3,000,000	$3,000,000	$3,000,000	Improve clinical documentation and coding.
Growth	14–Demand growth	$4,950,000	$5,692,500	$6,546,500	$7,528,000	Open new practices, and improve access to existing practices.
Forecasted gap		$36,500,000	$45,000,000	$51,000,000	$60,000,000	
Gap closure total		$35,360,000	$45,689,000	$56,800,000	$64,842,000	
Remaining gap		$1,140,000	–$689,000	–$5,800,000	–$4,842,000	

Note: DVT = deep vein thrombosis; LOS = length of stay; MGMA = Medical Group Management Association; VAP = ventilator-associated pneumonia.

The executive team then developed a multiyear gap closure strategy featuring the deployment of 11 expansive PI initiatives, including three initiatives focused exclusively on the physician practices division. If this plan succeeded, the organization would produce a positive operating margin by year 2.

Of note is that the strategy was built on assumptions of when benefits were expected to be achieved and an assumption that these savings would be sustained over time. For example, the labor productivity team forecasted a savings of 175 full-time equivalent staff in the first year. The $10.4 million savings would be sustained and accrue over subsequent years.

This example illustrates several dynamics of multiyear performance improvement:

- Short-term improvements are found primarily through a focus on labor productivity and nonlabor expenses.
- Revenue cycle improvements may generate substantial revenue gains in the short term as well, depending on the organization's current performance.
- These short-term initiatives are necessary but insufficient for closing large financial gaps over an extended period.
- Savings resulting from clinical utilization, off-quality, and portfolio improvements can be substantial, but they take longer to implement than revenue cycle improvements do. Benefits from the long-term initiatives generally accrue two to three years after launch.
- Revenue growth normally includes short-term tactical improvement and long-term strategic opportunities.

This example also illustrates how the 18 improvement levers align with the initiatives. The levers become the building blocks for the initiative teams to achieve the economic targets.

SEVEN PERFORMANCE IMPROVEMENT CATEGORIES

Improvement levers can be further categorized according to the focus of the intervention and the expected impact on the organization (exhibit 3.6). When categorized this way, the levers represent seven overall areas of improvement opportunity:

- Improving processes and facilities
- Aligning resources with demand

Exhibit 3.6: Seven Performance Improvement Categories

Improvement Category	Desired Outcomes	Improvement Levers
Improving processes and facilities	Improving the functional and cross-functional business processes and care environment factors that have the greatest impact on service, quality, and the cost of care	• Process improvement • Structural process improvement • Facilities optimization
Aligning resources with demand	Ensuring the right resources are available at the right time to fully meet the work demand	• Role and team redesign • Demand smoothing • Dynamic staffing • Demand regrouping
Leveraging the system	Exploiting the scale and efficiencies of a multientity health system	• Management restructuring • System rationalization • Service redeployment
Optimizing non-labor expenses	Ensuring supplies and other nonlabor expenses are effectively managed and deployed	• Nonlabor optimization
Improving quality and clinical utilization	Maximizing the clinical outcomes of patients who receive care while minimizing unnecessary care and costs and mitigating patient and organizational risk	• Utilization improvement • Off-quality improvement
Building top-line revenues	Growing top-line revenues through effective revenue management and strategic growth	• Demand growth • Revenue optimization
Optimizing the service portfolio	Building a strong service continuum through internal development and strategic sourcing	• Service outsourcing • Service divestment • Continuum realignment

- Leveraging the system
- Optimizing nonlabor expenses
- Improving quality and clinical utilization
- Building top-line revenues
- Optimizing the service portfolio

In part II, one chapter each is devoted to these categories, along with a detailed description of the associated improvement levers.

Healthcare Performance Improvement Levers

Regardless of the improvement model used, performance improvement initiatives typically include three generic, sequential components:

- An initial *assessment* of performance gaps and identification of improvement opportunities or performance that is below leadership's expectations or customers' requirements
- A *redesign* phase, in which a leader or team identifies root causes of low performance, generates alternative improvements or solutions to the performance issues, and identifies the best solutions going forward
- An *implementation* component, in which improvement interventions are put in place and leaders evaluate outcomes to see if the expected results are achieved

In chapter 2, a case is made for assessing the organization's core competencies and identifying systems and processes that need improvement to support process redesign and implementation. Using this information and additional quantitative analysis, the organization's leaders can identify targets, charter improvement teams, and initiate the redesign process.

The performance framework and 18 improvement levers are used in the redesign phase to focus leaders and teams on the few vital operational issues that are most common for their service or function. This narrowed focus enables groups to quickly inventory key business processes and the common operational issues associated with these processes. By focusing on the relevant subset of improvement levers, groups can identify operational solutions while avoiding prolonged brainstorming, analysis, and prioritization of ideas.

Part II is a review of the 18 performance improvement levers. A summary description of each is provided in appendix B.

CHAPTER 4

Improving Processes and Facilities

PROCESS IMPROVEMENT LEVERS are operational interventions executed either at the department or program level or across system entities. The scope and complexity of the process under review determines the time and resources required for redesign and implementation. Small process changes in a single department can be effected quickly, whereas complex, multifunctional processes can take months to redesign and involve many staff members.

Process improvement is a critical component of a healthcare organization's performance improvement (PI) strategy. Successful process improvement occurs when organizations

- focus on key business processes that have the greatest impact on patients and physicians,
- hardwire consumer feedback mechanisms and requirements into redesigned processes,
- engage key stakeholders in the evaluation and design process,
- use an improvement methodology that is understood by all involved,
- invest in training and technical support to ensure that leaders and teams use the appropriate improvement tools and methods at the right time, and
- avoid assigning process improvement teams to remedy every organizational issue—big and small.

The expansive industry adoption of total quality management, Lean, Six Sigma, and other methodologies underscores the applicability of process improvement to healthcare organizations. Healthcare providers deliver patient care—and do the work that supports it—through a network of clinical, administrative, and support processes. How well these processes are designed and executed generally determines the costs and quality of services provided to patients.

Performance improvement is largely concerned with changing work processes to yield increased value for customers. Operational improvement initiatives should begin with a focus on the organization's key processes and an understanding of how effectively services meet customer needs and demands. During the redesign phase, collaborative teams identify process gaps and improvement solutions. Crafting new processes is normally performed by collaborative teams, although much of the redesign fine-tuning occurs during implementation.

LEVER 1: PROCESS IMPROVEMENT

Healthcare leaders employ process improvement to strengthen the services and value provided to patients, families, physicians, and other stakeholder groups. These initiatives usually focus on improving one or more performance dimensions of a process, such as

- reducing the cycle time required for service completion;
- reducing errors, improving quality, and building consistency and reliability into work processes;
- minimizing the time spent on tasks that do not add value to the service performed;
- improving the cost-effective utilization of equipment, facilities, and supplies; and
- lowering the overall cost of service provision.

The services delivered by a health system are often complex, multistep processes involving numerous skill levels and departments. Room cleaning and setup in a surgery department provide just one example of the complexity in a process that is performed multiple times a day. Room turnover is a critical component of patient throughput for any surgery department. Shaving precious minutes off a room turnover process is a crucial lifesaving endeavor as well as a cost-saving effort.

The diagram in exhibit 4.1 presents the key components—the suppliers, inputs, processes, outputs, and customers (SIPOC)—of a typical surgical room turnover process. The main steps involved in room turnover include the cleaning of a room when a patient is moved or discharged and the setup of supplies and equipment for the next inpatient. Though seemingly straightforward, the process is fraught with complexity and unpredictability.

Customers and Outputs

Business processes are designed to produce *outputs*, in the form of services or products, to meet the needs of customers. Improving processes begins with identifying external and internal customer groups and understanding their needs and requirements for the services provided. These requirements are often referred to under the blanket term *voice of the customer (VOC)*. VOC helps define

- the process outputs, or what services should be produced;
- the product or service features;
- the timeliness of the service; and
- the desired cost and quality levels of the service.

Patient care services are intended to meet the needs of multiple internal and external customer groups. In the case of operating room (OR) turnover, several external customer groups, each with

Exhibit 4.1: Room Turnover and Setup in a Surgical Services Department

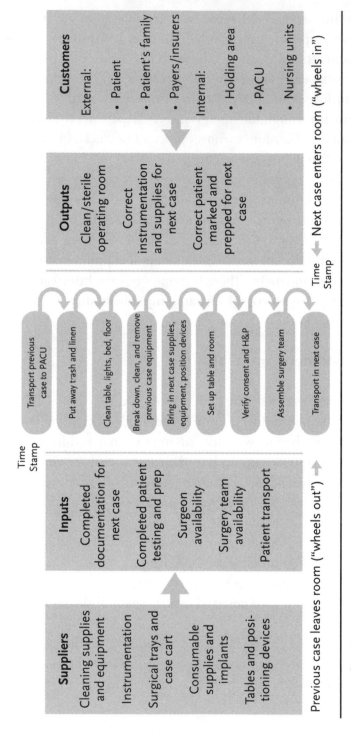

Suppliers

Cleaning supplies and equipment

Instrumentation

Surgical trays and case cart

Consumable supplies and implants

Tables and positioning devices

Inputs

Completed documentation for next case

Completed patient testing and prep

Surgeon availability

Surgery team availability

Patient transport

Time Stamp

Previous case leaves room ("wheels out")

- Transport previous case to PACU
- Put away trash and linen
- Clean table, lights, bed, floor
- Break down, clean, and remove previous case equipment
- Bring in next case supplies, equipment, position devices
- Set up table and room
- Verify consent and H&P
- Assemble surgery team
- Transport in next case

Time Stamp

Next case enters room ("wheels in")

Outputs

Clean/sterile operating room

Correct instrumentation and supplies for next case

Correct patient marked and prepped for next case

Customers

External:
- Patient
- Patient's family
- Payers/insurers

Internal:
- Holding area
- PACU
- Nursing units

Note: H&P = history and physical; PACU = post-acute care unit.

specific expectations, are involved. For example, patients and sur-geons require efficiency in the room turnover and setup processes to minimize delays and ensure that the room is sterile and contains the correct equipment and instruments for the upcoming surgery. Internal customers include staff in other sections of the surgery department and nursing staff on the medical–surgical unit whose work is affected by patient throughput in the OR.

Customer principles are equally applicable to ambulatory services. For example, when a physician orders an outpatient CT (computed tomography) scan for her patient, she and her office staff require specific service requirements, such as the following:

- Appointment access for patients
- Ease of scheduling
- Timeliness and thoroughness of results reporting
- Quality and reliability of the imaging staff
- Quality of and consultative access to the interpreting radiologist

Patients have similar service expectations of the CT department:

- Ease of appointment scheduling
- Sufficient parking and access to the imaging center
- Minimal waiting time to be seen
- Friendliness and helpfulness of the front-desk and technical staff
- Efficient and accurate insurance, billing, and payment processes

Suppliers and Inputs

Understanding a process also requires knowledge of the key *inputs* required to perform the service. Inputs include resources and condi-tions necessary to provide the service, such as the following:

- Sufficient staffing levels
- Available supplies and equipment
- Complete and timely information
- Facility capacity and access
- Patient access and availability

Surgery delays may occur as a result of factors relating to supplies and other inputs, such as the following:

- Missing or incomplete documentation for the next patient
- Additional presurgical testing
- Detained or delayed surgeons
- Missing patients (the next patient is not ready or is awaiting transportation from a nursing unit)

Process Measurement

Leaders must have systems in place to *measure* the current performance of a process. Most processes have several performance dimensions, requiring multiple metrics. In the previous CT services example, the imaging center manager should track the following metrics:

- Patient satisfaction
- Patient waiting time
- Scheduling availability (average days out to schedule patients)
- Referring physician satisfaction
- Direct cost and contribution margin per procedure
- Radiologist reporting turnaround time

When possible, the manager should compare these values to internal and external benchmarks to understand which dimensions of performance have improvement potential.

Process Evaluation and Improvement

After identifying key inputs and outputs, a leader may form an improvement team to document the steps that make up the process as it is currently, or is intended to be performed. Most process improvement teams use flowcharting techniques to document the sequential steps in a process. The most common tools used to document business processes are the following:

- *SIPOC diagram*—A high-level chart whose development often precedes the construction of a detailed flowchart. The SIPOC diagram documents suppliers, inputs, a process overview, outputs, and customers.
- *Flowchart*—A standardized process chart that provides a graphical representation of steps and sequence. It defines the starting and stopping points of the process and usually includes key decision points (depicted as diamonds) that lead to alternative workflows.
- *Swim lane diagram*—A type of flowchart that groups each process step according to the person or function responsible for its performance. A swim lane diagram is useful for sorting steps by time interval and illustrating simultaneously performed tasks.
- *Value stream map*—An advanced form of flowchart found frequently in Lean initiatives. A value stream map is used to highlight the degree of value that each step brings to a process. This approach is particularly beneficial for identifying opportunities to reduce waste and accelerate cycle time for work completion.

Teams use depictions of a process *as it currently is performed* to identify steps in the process that

- do not add value to customers or the completion of the process,

- are redundant with other steps,
- generate waste or underutilization of resources,
- increase the process cycle time because of delays, and
- create unnecessary handoffs or complexity.

Frequently, improvement teams use brainstorming to generate a list of potential factors that contribute to suboptimal performance. A cause-and-effect diagram can be used to summarize the primary and secondary causal factors. With additional data collection, a team can identify a subset of causal factors that most contribute to low performance.

Next, process improvement teams generate ideas and solutions—through brainstorming, benchmarking, and other methods—that address the primary causal factors. At this point, the team may employ trial runs, simulation modeling, or other techniques to test improvement interventions in advance of full implementation. From this work, the team documents the redesigned process as it is intended to be performed.

Process improvement should focus, in part, on addressing critical barriers or constraints to patients, materials, or information flow. Projects focused on discrete parts of a process can suboptimize the whole. For example, a quicker turnaround of CT scans for emergency patients may not relieve emergency department (ED) congestion if other care processes prevent earlier discharges or more timely inpatient admissions. High-value process improvement tackles those opportunities that represent removing or improving critical process constraints.

Implementation follows the design phase. During implementation, leaders monitor the performance of the redesigned workflow. The same process metrics are used to determine if the expected improvements have been realized. Process designs are often adjusted early in implementation on the basis of the initial lessons learned.

The following case study applies the principles of Lean and Six Sigma to the process of room turnover in a busy OR.

CASE EXAMPLE: PROCESS IMPROVEMENT—
SURGICAL ROOM TURNOVER

A large academic medical center needed to increase capacity in the OR to accommodate additional cases resulting from new surgeon recruitment. The executive team was specifically interested in adding cases during the core weekday hours of 7:00 a.m. to 5:00 p.m. Increasing capacity on weekends or at night was not desirable, as this option would incur added staffing and other incremental expenses. Additionally, project recommendations could not be tied to large-scale investments (e.g., building a new OR) because of limitations in available capital.

The hospital's executive leadership chartered five collaborative teams to address different factors affecting room utilization and surgical capacity. One team focused on the between-case turnover of surgery rooms with the goal of reducing the time between cases required to clean a room, set up for the next case, and bring the next patient to the OR suite. Current data revealed that the department consistently failed to achieve target turnaround times for most rooms and services, as shown in the table that follows.

Comparison of Target (per hospital policy) Versus Actual Surgery Room Turnover Time

Case Type	Target (minutes)	Actual Average (minutes)
Outpatient	20.0	29.6
Inpatient	40.0	43.8
Pediatric	30.0	33.6
Weighted average	25.2	35.2

On the basis of the organization's volume and mix of procedures, the difference between actual and targeted turnover time resulted in an additional five hours per weekday of unplanned room turnover time.

From these conclusions, the executive team developed a charter for a surgery room turnover team and recruited surgeons, clinical and operational staff, and department leadership to serve as members. The team leaders included three surgeons who were recognized by the surgical staff as having consistently favorable room turnover times.

The team was charged with achieving the following outcomes:

- Improve the weighted average room turnover time by at least ten minutes per case.
- Design new processes to consistently meet or exceed current turnover targets.
- Reduce case delays attributed to "room not ready" issues.
- Identify labor and nonlabor resource requirements.
- Assign and communicate roles and responsibilities.
- Reduce equipment-related delays.

The room turnover team met weekly for two hours over a six-week period using the define, measure, analyze, improve, and control (DMAIC) framework from Six Sigma methodology.

Setting Target Performance Levels: The Define and Measure Phases

In the initial meeting, the team reviewed available data to understand current room turnover performance by team, room, and surgeon. The team focused on process improvement issues related to room cleanup and setup activities occurring from "wheels-in to wheels-out," or the time spent between the point at which one patient is transported from the room and the arrival of the next patient.

Team members believed the organization could lower turnaround averages to levels below the targets set by department policy. This conclusion was supported by external benchmarks and the experiences of team members at other hospitals. The team recommended stretch goals for turnover according to type of patient case, as shown in the following list:

- Outpatient—15 minutes
- Inpatient—30 minutes
- Complex—45 minutes

On the basis of the department's mix of cases (outpatient, 52 percent; inpatient, 28 percent; complex, 20 percent), the weighted average target was 25.2 minutes.

Analysis and Findings: The Analyze Phase

As a starting point for the analysis phase, the team evaluated room turnover time by clinical service (exhibit 4.2). Data analysis revealed that room turnover time varied, in part, with the acuity of the service, with cardiothoracic surgery experiencing the longest turnover times. However, exceptions were seen, as orthopedics experienced below-average turnover times despite performing procedures that typically had demanding room setup requirements.

From this and other analysis of turnover data, the executive team concluded the following:

- Statistically significant turnover time differences were seen on the basis of specialty and patient type.
- The average turnover for an OR room did not vary considerably (two to three minutes) from month to month.
- Turnover times were consistently above the targets, indicating potential structural issues that drive high turnover times.

The team reviewed and updated existing process flowcharts for the entire perioperative throughput process. Team members analyzed

Exhibit 4.2: Average Surgery Room Turnover Time by Clinical Service

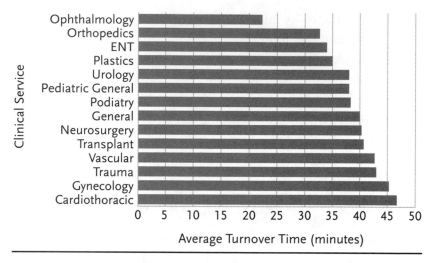

Note: ENT = ear, nose, and throat.

their assigned portion of the process and flagged steps where problems and issues occurred.

Next, the team leader facilitated a brainstorming exercise with the group to identify the causal factors of slow room turnover time. The results of this exercise were used to construct a detailed cause-and-effect diagram, also known as a fishbone diagram or an Ishikawa diagram (exhibit 4.3).

Some of the key conclusions reached from this exercise included the following:

- Many of the issues that generated case delays also drove high room turnover times. The department struggled with on-time starts for the first case of the day. At the time of the project, 47 percent of first-case starts began at least ten minutes later than scheduled. The turnover team addressed the portion of delays associated with room cleaning and setup.

Exhibit 4.3: Operating Room Turnover Cause-and-Effect Analysis

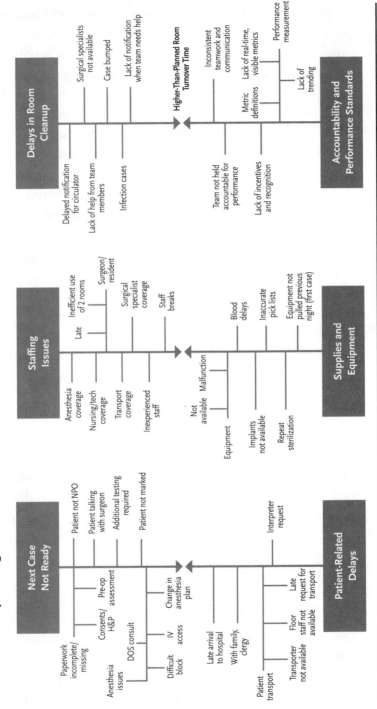

Note: DOS = day of surgery; H&P = history and physical; IV = intravenous; NPO = nil per os (nothing by mouth; i.e., patient did not adhere to NPO instructions).

- A portion of setup time delays was driven by the location of the OR with respect to other areas. For example, some rooms were located a significant distance from supply storage and central processing areas, resulting in lengthy staff travel times. Other rooms were situated far from the holding area, exacerbating patient transport time.
- Many delays were driven by the lack of equipment, particularly portable radiology equipment and microscopes.
- The team members spoke at length about the behavioral, competency, and motivational issues of staff and how these factors affected the efficiency of room turnover. From their perspectives, effective room turnover required teams to have
  - members who are skilled in their specialty and experienced with the equipment and setup;
  - clearly defined roles that were understood by all team members and performed in parallel with other tasks;
  - members with a supportive, cooperative attitude and a teamwork orientation; and
  - real-time turnover measures to motivate staff and track performance.
- The team members described the typical competitive nature of people who work in surgery programs, and how this competitive spirit should be leveraged in the department to improve performance. This leveraging could be accomplished, in part, by tracking and posting team turnover performance and recognizing and rewarding the top-performing teams.
- Since turnaround requirements are a function of both the type of case completed and the type of case to be set up, each event is unique. Only the surgeon and care team in the room have a fully informed understanding of what is required to complete the room turnover and should, therefore, have responsibility for setting turnover targets.

- Regarding specific roles and responsibilities for turnover, the team identified several critical issues:
  - Clarity about specific roles and responsibilities was lacking with many surgery teams.
  - Most team members performed turnover tasks in a sequential manner rather than in parallel with the work of other staff. This resulted in non-value-added waiting time at different points in the process.
  - The sharing of cleaning and setup responsibilities varied considerably from team to team, creating workload imbalance among team members.
  - Cleanup normally occurred once the first case vacated the room. The team believed cleanup should begin before the first case was transported to recovery.

The room turnover team next reviewed reasons for case delays. The group performed a Pareto analysis (Tague 2005) to identify the key factors causing delays and to determine the portion of delays attributed to room turnover issues (exhibit 4.4).

Eleven factors accounted for 80 percent of case delays. Approximately 40 percent of delays resulted from paperwork and anesthesia delays for the next case, which were addressed by a different team. The turnover team's work focused on the 20 percent of case delays caused by room-cleaning and setup issues. The team concluded that improving turnover would help lower case delays but would not remedy many of the delays in case starts.

The Improve Phase

The team formulated recommendations for improving the room turnover process. The recommendations were supported in part by industry best practices and other published benchmarking information and in part by the effectiveness of practices used by other internal teams.

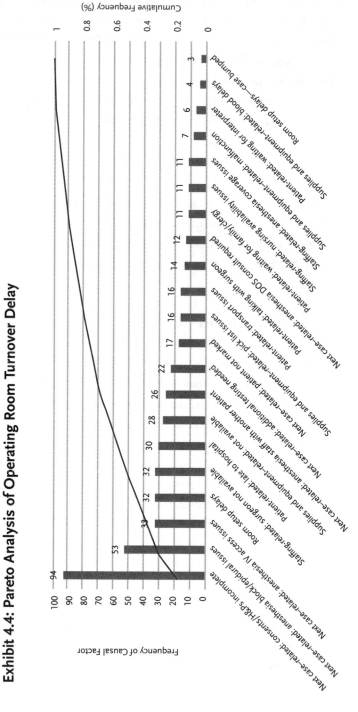

Exhibit 4.4: Pareto Analysis of Operating Room Turnover Delay

Cumulative Frequency (%)

Frequency of Causal Factor

Next case–related: consents/H&P's incomplete — 94
Next case–related: anesthesia block/epidural issues — 53
Next case–related: anesthesia IV access issues — 33
Room setup delays — 32
Staffing-related: surgeon not available — 32
Supplies and equipment–related: late to hospital — 30
Next case–related: anesthesia staff with another patient — 28
Next case–related: additional testing needed — 26
Supplies and equipment–related: patient not marked — 22
Patient–related: pick list issues — 17
Patient–related: transport issues — 16
Next case–related: anesthesia DOS consult required — 16
Patient–related: waiting for family/clergy — 14
Staffing-related: nursing availability issues — 12
Staffing-related: anesthesia coverage issues — 11
Supplies and equipment–related: malfunction — 11
Patient–related: waiting for interpreter — 11
Supplies and equipment–related: blood delays — 7
Room setup delays—case bumped — 6
4
3

Note: Analysis period is one month. DOS = day of surgery; H&P = history and physical; IV = intravenous.

Standardized Work

The team first applied standardized work principles to improve room turnover performance. A key aspect of the team's improvement effort was to define primary turnover roles and responsibilities for each member of the surgical team. Using a swim lane construct (exhibit 4.5), the group developed a proposed room turnover process to delineate sequenced task assignments by team role and demonstrate how these tasks should be performed in parallel with other tasks.

The new design moved selected tasks as early in the process as possible, including when the first patient is still in the OR. Some of the tasks occurring earlier in the process, along with their responsible parties, include the following:

- Anesthesiologist—complete anesthesia preoperative activities
- Surgical specialist—initiate cleaning tasks and bring in equipment
- Scrub technicians—clean instruments
- Circulator, or circulating nurse—complete documentation, charging, and other paperwork
- Surgeon—verify the next procedure, and ask for the next patient to be sent
- Vendor representative—make sure equipment is ready for the next case

Load Leveling

The revised process shown in the swim lane diagram assumes that all the personnel performing roles related to the case are available and present to assist with turnover. However, at times, fewer team members are available to assist, and other staff are directed to assist in completing tasks outside of their primary assignments. For example, surgical specialists are routinely delayed, occupied with cleaning other rooms or transporting patients, in which case others on the team, including surgeons, help with room cleanup and setup.

Exhibit 4.5: Swim Lane Diagram of Proposed Surgical Room Turnover Process

Role	Closing Timeout and Case Completion				Room Turnover and Setup			
	-30 min	-20 min	-10 min	Wheels Out (0)	+10 min	+15 min	+20 min	Wheels In
Surgeon	Specify what we just did and what we are about to do.							
		Ask if next patient has been sent for.						
		Verify next procedure.						
		Perform closure/provide instructions for closure.						
		Perform final counts.						
				Assist with transport, if needed.				
					Meet and mark next patient.			
					Make sure H&P is up-to-date; verify consent.			
						Talk with patient/family.		
							Assist with transport, if needed.	
						Document coding, billing, and operative notes.		

(continued)

(continued from previous page)

Exhibit 4.5: Swim Lane Diagram of Proposed Surgical Room Turnover Process

Role		Closing Timeout and Case Completion				Room Turnover and Setup		
	−30 min	−20 min	−10 min	Wheels Out (0)	+10 min	+15 min	+20 min	Wheels In
Anesthesia staff			Wake up patient.	Transport patient to PACU (stay in PACU if nurse is not available)/perform sign-out.				
			Move patient to stretcher.					
					Assist with room turnover (outpatient).			
						Sign in patient (CRNA).		
						Pick up and prepare medications.		
						Check anesthesia equipment.		
						Sign in patient (holding).		
							Transport patient to room.	
Circulating nurse	Call for next case.	Verify implant for next case with coordinator.						

(continued)

(continued from previous page)

Exhibit 4.5: Swim Lane Diagram of Proposed Surgical Room Turnover Process

	Closing Timeout and Case Completion				Room Turnover and Setup			
Role	–30 min	–20 min	–10 min	Wheels Out (0)	+10 min	+15 min	+20 min	Wheels In
			Call surgical specialist (for inpatient, call anesthesia technician).					
				Lead room turnover.				
				Record time stamp (wheels out).				
			Perform final count.				Declare room is ready.	
			Complete final documentation, complete chargeables, turn in paperwork to front desk, record time stamp.					
					Meet with CRNA and patient, sign patient into holding, assist scrub staff to open, get gowned.			
					Bring in equipment, instrumentation, and positioning devices.			
							Assist with transport, if needed.	

(continued)

Exhibit 4.5: Swim Lane Diagram of Proposed Surgical Room Turnover Process

Role	Closing Timeout and Case Completion				Room Turnover and Setup			
	−30 min	−20 min	−10 min	Wheels Out (0)	+10 min	+15 min	+20 min	Wheels In
Scrub nurse/ technician			Perform final count.			Put away trash and linen, sponges in biohazard bags.		
			Clean equipment and instruments; move them out of room.		Assist with room turnover.			
					Check case cart; open and get gowned.			
					Bring in equipment, instruments, and positioning devices; set up table; expedite counting.			
Surgical specialist			Clean room, starting with table, lights, trash, linen, bed, floor (C. *dif* infection takes longer to clean for).					
			Bring in equipment and instrumentation, positioning devices, and beds.		Bring in equipment and instrumentation, positioning		Assist with transport, if needed.	

Note: Example relates to a 20-minute turnover. C. *dif* = *Clostridium difficile*; CRNA = certified registered nurse anesthetist; H&P = history and physical; PACU = post-acute care unit.

The department previously scheduled first-case starts for all rooms at 7:00 a.m. Most first cases conclude between 9:30 a.m. and 10:00 a.m., creating a spike in rooms requiring turnover. The first-case start improvement team recommended adopting a staggered start schedule for the first cases in the morning to level out workloads during the morning hours. This recommendation had the added benefit of leveling demand for room turnover during the mid-mornings for the surgical specialists and others involved in room turnover.

Staff Breaks

Staff breaks, when taken between cases, can affect the ability of surgery teams to turn rooms over in a timely manner. The department lacked protocols for defining when breaks should occur. The room turnover team recommended the following:

- Staff should avoid between-case breaks that affect room turnover.
- Surgery team breaks should occur during procedures for all areas (ideally at the beginning or middle of cases). The exceptions were joint replacement cases and other procedures in which room entry is controlled as a precaution to prevent infections.
- Surgeons should be the only team members to take breaks between cases.
- Staggered schedules for surgical specialists' breaks should be adopted.

Technology Enabler

Concurrent with the work of the turnover team, the hospital implemented RFID (radio-frequency identification) technology in the surgery department. The tagging system is used to track equipment, supplies, and staff on a real-time basis and support improved communication among staff members. For room turnover, the team recommended employing the technology to

- record wheels-in and wheels-out times using a programmable button on the circulator's badge;
- send notifications from the circulator to the surgical specialists (also using a badge button) to eliminate most telephone notification calls;
- locate equipment and supplies using real-time tracking to dramatically reduce time spent searching for those items; and
- use badge buttons to notify the department when a team requires extra assistance with a room turnover.

Preference Cards

Preference cards are procedure-specific lists of surgical instruments and supply items reflecting the preference of the surgeon. (While physical cards are uncommon now, the terminology is still used.) Outdated preference cards can contribute to delays in room setup. At the time of the study, 75 percent of preference cards were out-of-date at the hospital. This absence of accurate information resulted in start-time delays when surgical instrument trays contained unnecessary items or incorrect items. Missing items must be located and frequently require flash sterilization. The team formulated several recommendations for updating preference cards for high-volume procedures.

Visual Cues

The team believed that visual devices, including postings of process goals, should be in place to support the new turnover process. The team recommended the following process changes:

- During the timeout phase of the first case of the day, the surgeon should determine and communicate the expected turnover time for the next case.
- The circulating nurse should record the target timeout and expected completion time on the whiteboard so everyone

on the team understands the target wheels-in time for the next case.

- The circulating nurse should record a time stamp for "room ready." This additional measure would enable the department to track room completion delays separately from other delays that affect turnover times.
- Digital clocks should be used in the OR as an aid to count down the time to room completion.

The group also recommended using readily visible goal-tracking devices to track and communicate turnover performance by surgery team. As a result, the OR directors began posting graphical summaries of performance for all department staff to view. The top-performing teams were recognized and rewarded for their efforts.

Behavioral Changes

Finally, the team identified behavioral changes needed to meet the department's room turnover goals. Specifically, the team recommended the following:

- Communicate the new, expected room turnover standards.
- Update the room turnover policy and procedure documentation to reflect the new targets.
- Establish a standard definition of *turnover* that is understood by all stakeholders.
- Communicate roles and responsibilities, and provide training as required.
- Recognize and reward high-performing teams.
- Employ the department's internal performance improvement team to address ongoing process and behavioral issues.

Estimation of Economic Benefit

The work of the room turnover team demonstrated that the organization had the potential to improve turnover by 30 to 40 percent. The combined improvements in turnover processes reduced the weighted average turnover time to 20–25 minutes. This decrease represented an improvement of 10 to 15 minutes per case. The combined process and system changes from the turnover team and other groups working on surgical services issues freed additional capacity, resulting in an estimated 15 to 21 additional surgery cases per week, representing $4.0 to $5.5 million in additional annual contribution margin.

LEVER 2: STRUCTURAL PROCESS IMPROVEMENT

The preceding case example demonstrates process improvement applied in a single department. Structural process improvement focuses on improving cross-functional and cross-entity business processes. In a healthcare system, key business processes represent activities that

- are most visible to patients and have a significant impact on service and patient satisfaction,
- are instrumental to efficient patient throughput and coordination of care across departments and care sites,
- drive much of the operating costs in a health system, and
- can have a direct impact on clinical quality outcomes.

Some examples of common health system business processes include the following:

- Ambulatory care
  - Patient access and scheduling
  - Referrals to specialists and hospital services
  - Professional billing
  - Outpatient service delivery
- Acute care
  - Patient admissions and preadmissions processes
  - Perioperative throughput

- ED patient throughput
- Outpatient scheduling and registration
- Bed control and room turnover
- Supply chain management
- Patient discharge processes
- Patient charging and billing
- Post-acute care
  - Acute care patient transfers to post-acute providers
  - Home care service delivery
  - Patient charging and billing
- Revenue cycle
  - Procedure scheduling
  - Insurance preauthorization
  - Patient finance education and counseling
  - Provider education
  - Payment denial management
  - Payer relations

The tools and approaches for structural process improvement are similar to those used in functional or process improvement. The added scope and complexity, however, require teams to address a broader range of issues. Thus, structural process improvement takes additional time and involves a greater number of people. For example, a team focused on improving the inpatient discharge and transfer process may include the following personnel:

- Case managers
- Social workers
- Nurse managers
- Hospitalists
- Bed management staff
- Patient transportation staff or volunteers
- Home care managers
- The director of long-term care services
- Health information management staff

- Information services staff
- Internal PI consultants

Frequently, a core team assigns components of the process to subteams to review performance and formulate recommendations for improvement. Subteams help accelerate the improvement process and engage an overall larger group of individuals in the process.

Patient Throughput

Healthcare systems focus much of their structural process improvement efforts on enhancing cross-functional service coordination and patient throughput. In an integrated health system (exhibit 4.6), structural processes are the primary links between system entities that follow a patient's progression of care.

The goal of throughput improvement is to design processes that move patients seamlessly from one care setting to the next. Effective patient throughput

- places patients in the right care setting at the right time,
- frees up service capacity to accommodate additional patients,
- lowers fixed and variable operating expenses by reducing the cost of holding patients who are waiting for services or are waiting to be discharged home,
- improves patient satisfaction (Kane et al. 2015; Parker and Marco 2014), and
- improves clinical outcomes (Tsai, Oray, and Jha 2015; Singer et al. 2011; Chalfin et al. 2007).

Patient throughput is also critical for managing the length of stay (LOS) for inpatients. Reimbursement for acute care has shifted largely to a per case basis. Hospitals have a strong financial incentive to manage LOS, minimize unnecessary patient days, and appropriately place patients in post-acute services.

Exhibit 4.6: Throughput Processes in an Integrated Health System

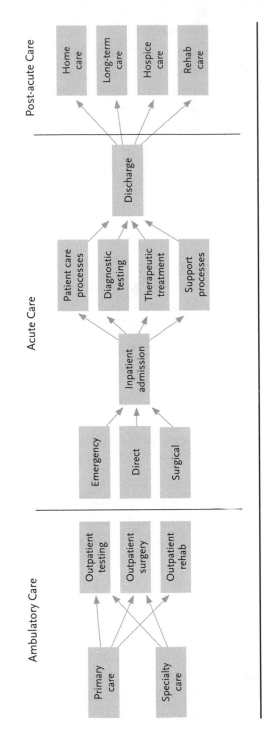

High-performing healthcare systems focus significant attention and resources on improving patient throughput. These organizations adopt and build high-performing, evidence-based practices into patient care and fully engage physicians in throughput improvement initiatives. Such initiatives aim to improve each component of the throughput process as follows:

- Patient admission
    - Direct admission procedures are well-defined, thorough, and communicated effectively to admitting physicians.
    - Physicians rarely admit patients who do not meet clinical criteria for inpatient or observation status.
    - A patient admitted in the ED or transferred from recovery or critical care is almost always admitted or transferred within one hour of disposition.
    - Physicians plan the potential discharge date with the patient at the time of admission and work with the care coordinators to meet or adjust the date as appropriate.
- Case management
    - Interdisciplinary rounds occur daily with the case managers and clinical care providers.
    - Case managers and the patient's nurse review patients on observation status every four to six hours.
    - Case managers review the status of all ED patients prior to admission as inpatients or for observation and all other patients prior to or within 12 hours of admission.
    - A utilization committee meets regularly to review data, monitor concurrent medical necessity compliance processes, participate in peer review processes, and identify improvement opportunities.

- An effective denial management process is in place, and finance personnel and case managers meet routinely to identify improvement opportunities.
- Patients who represent outliers above a certain day or dollar threshold are monitored by an executive team with the authority to influence discharge processes.
- Inpatient care
  - Physicians consistently communicate the patient's plan of care to other care providers.
  - Physicians adhere to available protocols or clinical pathways.
  - Physicians attend daily interdisciplinary clinical team meetings.
  - Hospitalists lead patient care planning, following patients from admission to discharge with assessments every 4 to 12 hours depending on patient needs.
  - All inpatients are assigned a targeted LOS, which is shared with caregivers and patients and their families.
  - Specialists consistently provide timely consultations and reporting.
- Patient discharge
  - Physicians enter discharge orders in the early morning of or the night before discharge, so inpatients may depart by 11:00 a.m. or within an hour of their designated discharge time.
  - Hospitalists, residents, and attending physicians are available to prepare paperwork for early morning discharge orders.
  - Representatives from home health, rehabilitation, ambulance, and other outside agencies are available and aligned with patient flow goals.
  - Prescriptions, durable medical equipment, and all other services are arranged prior to discharge.

- Throughput measurement
  - Avoidable stay days are tracked daily and improvement opportunities identified.
  - Key patient flow measures (ED wait time, backlog for critical care beds, ED diversions) are regularly collected in a dynamic, anticipatory measurement system.
  - Bed capacity is measured and analyzed for trends by hour of day, day of week, or season. The information is communicated routinely to executive staff and operational areas such as patient access, nursing services, and environmental services to manage and improve throughput and capacity.
  - LOS data by unit, physician, and diagnosis are continuously collected and shared with clinicians.
- Technology support
  - The organization has information systems in place to collect bed utilization, capacity, patient tracking, and throughput management data.
  - The organization's electronic health record supports effective clinical documentation, order entry, and clinical pathway adherence.

Patient throughput initiatives require a structured evaluation process and an effective approach for engaging physicians and other clinicians. The following case is an example of a multidisciplinary improvement team aiming to enhance the throughput efficiency of patients admitted from an ED.

CASE EXAMPLE: CROSS-FUNCTIONAL PROCESS IMPROVEMENT

A large tertiary hospital was experiencing significant delays in placing critical care patients admitted from the ED. At the time, the

Level I trauma center was seeing an average of 400 patients per day. Patient flow challenges frequently occurred throughout the facility, but senior leaders were particularly concerned about ED bottlenecks. ED length of stay for patients admitted to the medical intensive care unit (MICU) averaged 8.5 hours, exceeding national averages and best practices by a factor of two or greater.

The organization's executive leadership assigned a multidisciplinary team to evaluate the admissions process and set a goal of reducing the average LOS for admitted patients to 4.0 hours. This team was sponsored by the vice president of medicine and included 12 team members representing

- ED leadership;
- physicians from the ED, the trauma unit, and the hospitalist department;
- nursing staff from the ED, MICU, and pulmonary step-down unit;
- case management staff;
- admissions and bed board staff;
- information services data analysis staff; and
- operations excellence staff.

The team met three or four times per week over a three-week period to develop and adopt a rapid-cycle improvement process. Each meeting was scheduled for four hours. Team leaders employed a *kaizen* improvement framework (Graban and Swartz 2014) supported by the principles of

- value stream mapping,
- just-in-time Lean training,
- forms of waste,
- pull systems,
- single-piece flow,
- mistake-proofing,
- teamwork, and
- standardized work.

As an initial step, the team constructed a value stream map of the ED admissions process to the ICU. At a high level, the process worked as depicted in exhibit 4.7.

By documenting the current process, the team revealed the number of handoffs occurring among individuals, each with the potential for delay or miscommunication. Additionally, the patient admission

---

Exhibit 4.7: High-Level View of Emergency Department (ED) Patient Admission Process

Patient assessed and stabilized by ED physician.

↓

ED physician requests ED nurse to instruct ED clerk to send intensive care unit (ICU) bed request to bed coordinator.

↓

Bed coordinator calls medical ICU (MICU) charge nurse to determine bed availability.

↓

MICU charge nurse assesses bed availability status and apprises bed coordinator of when a bed will be available.

↓

Bed coordinator calls ED clerk to apprise of bed availability.

↓

ED clerk calls central transport to request patient transfer.

↓

ED nurse calls MICU and gives report on patient.

↓

Both ED nurse and transport technician accompany patient to MICU.

↓

ED physician conducts phone handoff to intensivist or critical care physician assistant.

---

workup was shown to vary by ED physician. Many members of the ED medical staff believed some critical patients could be better stabilized under their care than in the ICU. Some ED physicians were also concerned about turning over a patient to a MICU intensivist before completing a full diagnosis of the patient.

On the basis of an analysis of ED and census data, the team concluded that the shortage of MICU beds was a primary factor in the high ED length of stay for patients awaiting admission. The shortage of ICU beds could be attributed, in part, to delays in moving ICU patients to step-down units. Step-down beds were restricted by the high number of discharges occurring after daytime hours. The team concluded that responsibility for clinical management of step-down patients was lacking. Oversight was shared by multiple hospitalists who only saw step-down patients once daily, resulting in delays with discharge orders.

As a next step, the team identified metrics and information deemed critical to understanding the patient throughput process and its performance. Examples of these indexes included average time to triage, average time to see a physician, radiology and laboratory services turnaround time, and boarding time in the ED.

Introducing Idealized Design to Lean

As a basis for redesigning the patient admissions and bed placement processes, the team conducted a benchmarking survey of three other healthcare organizations to identify high-performing practices. The team leaders also conducted an idealized design (Ackoff, Magidson, and Addison 2006) exercise, which involves developing an inspiring vision of how a process should work perfectly. Steps in the exercise are as follows:

1. Identifying ideals, objectives, and goals
2. Designing the system that team members would want if they could start fresh

3. Developing that system in the constraints of
   a. technological feasibility,
   b. operational viability, and
   c. staff capability of learning and adapting

Using this approach, the team divided into four groups, each with three members. Working independently, the groups were tasked with answering the question: "If you could design an ED admissions process from scratch, how would you design it?" They reported their results to the full team, with the outcome that each team produced diverse ideas and process attributes. Many ideas were based on the Lean principles of pull systems, waste reduction, and standardized work.

The team identified the following desired improvement elements:

- We want a pull system throughout the patient stay, from presentation to discharge.
- Time spent while any patient waits in an inappropriate level of care is waste, and we want to avoid expending that wasted time.
- We want to handle each transfer only once. Multiple requests for beds, transporters, and handover meetings should be eliminated.
- MICU, ED, and step-down units will work together as a team to ensure that the patient always receives the right level of care (right patient, right bed).
- The procedures will be standardized and executed consistently on every shift.
- We will practice the Plan-Do-Check-Act approach to improvement, making process enhancements on a continuous basis.

Team members voted on the ideas and attributes from the idealized design exercise and incorporated the highest-ranking ideas into a future-state process map. The following design elements were translated into a new future state and practice:

- When an ED physician reaches the conclusion that a patient will require ICU care, the ICU is notified and a critical care nurse and MICU physician assistant (PA) immediately report to the ED to take charge of the patient.
- Face-to-face handoffs occur simultaneously between the ED nurse and critical care nurse or the ED attending physician and the MICU PA.
- The MICU team of nurse and PA is responsible to care for the patient and ensure that a bed in the MICU is readied. Until the patient is moved, the team remains with the patient in the ED. The patient is already "owned" by the ICU, regardless of location, even if she is still in the ED.
- ED staff provide any emergency assistance as necessary, but their time is largely freed up to manage other emergency patients.
- Medical accountability for patients in step-down beds has been redefined and rounding on these patients established twice per day, resulting in the easing of bed capacity bottlenecks.
- Patients with certain diagnoses or treatment requirements should be sent directly to the MICU. These include diabetic ketoacidosis, gastrointestinal bleeding that meets specified criteria, hypotension when on vasopressors, and intubation.
- An ED transporter has been designated for critical patients.

Results

To finalize the design, the team conducted a pilot of the new processes. During the 30-day pilot, ED length of stay for all critical care patients decreased from 6.45 hours to 3.61 hours. In the months following full implementation, the ED length of stay for critically ill patients was sustained at a 35 percent reduction. In addition, the overall hospital LOS for these patients decreased, and the total cost of care was reduced.

These outcomes could not have been achieved without the integration of Lean and idealized design principles. The design process created a safe environment for leaders and team members to articulate a progressive vision of perfect patient care. The kaizen format provided structure for the work, and Lean thinking pointed team members toward the operational ideals of no waste and smooth flow.

LEVER 3: FACILITY OPTIMIZATION

The physical layout of a facility is a prime factor in the flow of staff, patients, equipment, and supplies within and between departments. Facility and work area design factors can facilitate or limit effective operational performance. Poor workspace design adversely affects staff productivity because of

- increased travel time for staff within and between work areas,
- increased time for patient transport,
- increased time searching for and transporting supplies and equipment,
- lack of space to perform work or collaborate with other staff,
- lack of capacity to accommodate existing or additional caseloads,
- poor patient throughput resulting in delays and non-value-added work, and
- increased response time for services that support patient care (e.g., testing, therapies, pharmacy, meal delivery, room cleaning).

Many hospital facilities evolve over time, with new expansions pieced together with older buildings. Organizations with restricted capital operate in buildings that are 40 years old or older that were configured on the basis of outdated assumptions regarding patient volumes and care delivery processes.

Recently, the confluence of health reform, reimbursement changes, and advancements in technology has begun to transform medicine and the facilities that support care delivery. This discussion of facility optimization addresses common facility-related issues that collaborative teams often encounter as part of process improvement work. They mainly pertain to changes that have been effected for short-term benefit without the long-term considerations that come with significant redesign or capital investment. Large-scale facility transformation, while not covered in this book, will also be necessary for most health systems over the ensuing decades and will be a key determinant of long-term operational performance.

Facility optimization pertains to interventions that alter the space and configuration of a department or building to improve work performance. The scale of these changes can vary from large building programs and renovations to the reorganization of a small workspace in a department.

Facility Design

When evaluating processes and throughput, improvement teams should consider the following dimensions of facility design at a minimum:

- *Capacity*. Do we have sufficient functional space to accommodate workload requirements?
- *Proximity*. Are the resources and services most needed to perform work in a department located nearby?

- *Workflow and patient access.* Are facilities laid out in a manner that ensures the effective flow of patients, staff, and materials through the system?
- *Orderliness.* Is our department or work area clean, free of clutter, and organized?
- *Safety and security.* Do our facilities support a safe environment for patients, staff, and visitors?
- *Experience.* Do our facilities enhance the experience of patients and visitors and promote a strong brand in the market?

Each of these dimensions is explored in detail in the paragraphs that follow.

Capacity

Healthcare organizations must have sufficient space and facilities to meet current and future demand. Caregivers require adequate space and appropriate structure to accommodate patients and visitors, provide care, engage and interact with other staff, and have ready access to supplies and equipment. Insufficient capacity impedes productivity by restricting caseload and patient throughput, resulting in lowered staff utilization, unhappy physicians, and potential revenue losses. Additionally, lack of storage space leads to increased staff travel time to retrieve supplies and equipment from remote sites.

Clinical workspace, such as OR suites, ED rooms, and acute care rooms, must be plentiful and of the appropriate type and size to meet the demand and mix of patients and cases. Acute care services, for example, must have sufficient capacity for the following types of rooms:

- Routine medical–surgical
- Intensive care
- Telemetry monitoring

- Isolation
- Labor and delivery
- Recovery
- Observation

Similar requirements apply to ambulatory settings. Physician practices, for example, must have facilities that accommodate peak demand for waiting areas, examination and treatment rooms, and storage and space for front-office staff and functions.

Space planning and allocation is a related dimension of capacity management. Functional programming is most often used by architects to determine space requirements when planning new buildings. However, it is also a useful tool for assessing existing facilities to determine areas that are over- and underresourced with respect to space.

Functional programming begins with forecasting projected workload volumes, such as patient days, hours of surgery, and number of cases. Planners use forecasts to predict peak workload demands that must be accommodated by the new facility. This demand is then applied to industry benchmark standards for space requirements to calculate the total space required for a department. Projections are calculated according to the type of space, such as patient care, office space, storage, hallways, and common areas.

Facility capacity constraints are often symptomatic of suboptimal patient throughput and workflow. When evaluating capacity issues in patient care areas such as emergency services, inpatient nursing, and surgery, healthcare leaders should determine whether throughput process improvements can reduce the demand for facility expansion. For example, an ED struggling with case turnover has longer LOS than benchmarks and frequently operates at full capacity. Patients awaiting discharge or admission unnecessarily occupy ED rooms, producing increased waiting times for new patients. At first glance, leaders might conclude that the department requires additional rooms, when the real issue is the need to improve patient throughput.

Excess capacity can also be problematic. Too much space can increase staff and patient travel time and increase maintenance and cleaning expenses. In addition, an overabundance of space for one department can result in a space shortage for another program.

Health systems need to be able to expand or contract facility capacity in response to seasonal demand variation. This ability is particularly important with inpatient bed capacity. Some organizations flex inpatient bed capacity using seasonal units. In these cases, leaders increase capacity by designating units that are opened when demand spikes and closed during times of low demand. The advantages of using a seasonal unit approach are as follows:

- It disrupts a limited number of areas.
- Accountability for seasonality is given to specific individuals.
- Predictability in staffing and scheduling is improved.
- Support and ancillary staff are better able to plan their support resources.

The ability to use the seasonal approach depends on the magnitude of the volume increase and the availability of units and beds that can be opened and closed.

The changing nature of patient care requires that facilities be flexible in the face of evolving demand. The traditional acute care–centric hospital design is being transformed as a result of the continued transitioning of medical care from acute to ambulatory and home-based services. Health systems will increasingly require flexible workspace design to expand or contract capacity in patient care and other service areas.

Proximity
Healthcare facility design should account for key functional adjacencies that are critical for optimal service provision to patients. Numerous examples can be seen in hospitals of interdependent

functions that should be in proximity to each other. These include the following:

- Laboratory and emergency services
- Surgery and sterile processing
- Patient registration and preadmission testing
- Respiratory therapy and intensive care

Architectural planning often includes proximity charting to identify locational requirements for medical and support programs and services. This information is used to determine where departments and functions should be located in a new facility. Specifically, proximity charts help determine the minimum distance requirements between departments and functions, often defined as high, medium, and not required.

Proximity principles are applicable to departments and smaller work areas. For example, supplies and equipment should be located near areas where they are used most frequently. Lack of proximity increases the time staff spend looking for supplies and equipment. Poor functional placement can also increase travel and transport time for patients moving between departments.

To resolve this issue when facility redesign or the building of facility extensions is not feasible, in some instances, a combination of centralization and decentralization may be used. For example, respirator storage may be located in or adjacent to the ICU or postanesthesia care unit if the respiratory therapy department is not in close proximity.

Workflow and Patient Access

Healthcare facilities should be designed to enable the effective flow of patients throughout the system. Facility planning must account for accessibility, sufficient capacity, and logical workflow that enhances the experience for patients. For example, a patient who arrives at a hospital for an outpatient imaging procedure expects

- a convenient location with geographical proximity to the patient's home;
- ample parking;
- signage and other wayfinding devices to locate the outpatient registration area;
- sufficient waiting area space;
- sufficient capacity in the medical imaging department to accommodate volume, thereby preventing long waiting times; and
- logical flow and structural setup for patient checkout.

Workflow is further supported by the availability of elevators, pneumatic tube systems, and other facility components that aid patients and visitors and support the work of physicians and hospital staff.

Orderliness

Facility design can also pertain to the design and condition of an individual's workspace or to small departmental work areas. The Lean methodology of the five Ss, described in the following list, provides a useful framework for setting up and maintaining effective workspaces (Chalice 2007, 80–82):

- *Sort*. Remove supplies, equipment, and other resources that are not necessary or are used rarely in the work of the department or function.
- *Straighten*. Make sure necessary resources (supplies, equipment, staff) can be located quickly when needed.
- *Shine*. Keep the work area clean and equipment well maintained.
- *Standardize*. Place every resource in a standard location.
- *Sustain*. Maintain consistency in the workspace environment.

Many healthcare organizations use the five-S principles to improve materials management and storage systems. Organized storage of supplies and equipment can

- reduce staff time required to locate supplies and equipment;
- reduce supply loss or expiration;
- reduce errors associated with the use of supplies;
- minimize the presence of unnecessary inventory;
- free up needed space; and
- maintain an orderly, safe environment for staff and patients.

Experience, Safety, and Security

Healthcare facilities should create an aesthetically appealing environment for patients, families, physicians, and staff. Pleasing environments are characterized by the following:

- Aesthetically appealing facilities that promote a noise-free, healing environment for patients
- Logical facility design and layout that facilitates the efficient flow of patients and visitors supported by effective signage and other wayfinding systems
- Facilities that provide designated family space in the patient room and family support space outside the patient room
- Facilities designed in a manner that promotes a safe, secure environment for patients, families, physicians, and staff

Facilities can significantly affect the patient experience and influence satisfaction scores. For physicians and staff, appealing work areas can enhance productivity and improve satisfaction.

Capital Equipment

Healthcare facilities require capital equipment to deliver patient care, conduct diagnostic services, and support administrative and nonpatient care services. Capital equipment investment in a health system is driven largely by a few key departments, including the following:

- *Surgical services*—electrosurgical equipment, autoclaves, tables, portable imaging equipment, microscopes, anesthesia equipment
- *Medical imaging*—CT, magnetic resonance imaging, and positron emission tomography scanners; ultrasound machines; nuclear medicine; and interventional radiology equipment
- *Laboratory*—diagnostic equipment and centrifuges
- *Cardiac services*—cardiac catheterization laboratory, electrophysiology lab, electrocardiogram equipment
- *Patient care*—patient beds, intravenous equipment, respirators, telemetry

Capital investment is ongoing, driven by the need to replace obsolete equipment, access new technologies, and accommodate the needs and preferences of physicians and patients. Most hospitals field capital requests that far exceed available funding. For this reason, organizations should have a formal capital requisition process in place that provides information and justification for the investment. Justification should be based on financial return on investment, quality and standard of care, increased market share capture, and other factors.

In addition to initial investment expense, equipment requires ongoing maintenance and support to remain functional and minimize downtime. Therefore, supply chain management should include the optimization of capital equipment use, taking into consideration the full life-cycle costs of equipment.

From a PI perspective, healthcare organizations should institute effective processes and systems to ensure that providers have the right equipment at the right time for serving patients. Capital equipment management systems should include the following components:

- An effective multiyear capital planning process for functional areas that enables leadership to proactively schedule and sequence major capital investments.
- Consistent protocols for requesting and evaluating proposed capital investments. Justification for investment should identify
  - safety and other patient care risks associated with maintaining current technologies,
  - indirect costs, and
  - potential revenue impact.
- Accurate asset tracking systems.
- Scrutiny of capital requests for replacement of equipment.
- Standardization of equipment across the system to improve pricing leverage with suppliers.

Facility issues are an important factor in healthcare service provision because

- facilities have a significant impact on processes and workflows;
- facility issues have a particularly high impact on supply chain management;
- facilities enhance or detract from an effective care environment, and they heavily influence patient satisfaction; and
- facilities play a primary role in shaping the organization's brand with patients and the community, and as such they should be an area of focus in PI initiatives.

Facility Issues and Performance Improvement Teams

Particularly in terms of the final point in the preceding list, collaborative teams often encounter and must address facility issues as part of process improvement. Specific facility issues vary with the type of team. Depending on the area of focus, a team leader should instruct team members to consider the following facility-related questions:

- *Productivity teams.* What facility issues are driving increased staffing costs and low productivity?
- *Growth teams.* What facility investments are necessary to grow patient volumes, expand markets, and grow revenues?
- *Portfolio teams.* How can we repurpose current facilities to strengthen the organization's service portfolio?
- *Nonlabor teams.* What facility changes can be made to improve supply chain processes and inventory management?
- *Throughput teams.* What facility changes are needed to improve the flow of patients through the care continuum?

Process and facility improvements are foundational to a comprehensive PI strategy. Breakthrough improvements in quality and operational performance are often enabled through redesigning work processes and enhancing facilities. This redesign work may precede the application of other PI levers. Process redesign, for example, can be critical to supporting leaders in redesign work teams and roles. In other cases, process and facility redesign follows decisions regarding large structural- or portfolio-level changes.

CHAPTER 5

Aligning Resources with Demand

HIGH-PERFORMING ORGANIZATIONS CONTINUOUSLY seek to improve the balance of resources to workload while delivering high-quality care and service. Sustaining high operational performance and productivity requires leaders to consistently deploy the right level and mix of resources (e.g., labor, supplies, equipment) at the right time to meet service demands. Achieving demand alignment can be challenging for many managers. To perform effectively, leaders must

- understand the demand dynamics for their services and how workload is distributed over time,
- have predictive systems and contingency plans in place to anticipate future spikes and declines in demand,
- maintain staffing resource flexibility to enable responsiveness to workload changes, and
- schedule work in a manner that minimizes workload variation and maintains workload balance across shifts and days of the week.

The improvement levers covered in this chapter are strategies for ensuring successful alignment of labor and other resources to variable workload demands. Specifically, they address key areas associated with the following activities:

- Controlling the demand for labor by streamlining key business processes
- Managing the demand for services with the goal of reducing variability in workload
- Designing roles and jobs that leverage the collective skills of the work group while maintaining staffing flexibility
- Leveraging this flexibility to optimally schedule staffing resources to meet the demand and deliver service-level requirements

Successfully aligning resources to demand is beneficial to all who are involved. For example:

- Patients receive the right service at the right time delivered by staff with the right skills and training to do so.
- Physicians' workdays are more predictable than when resource and demand are out of balance, and physicians have the right resources available to support their work.
- Staff benefit from predicable work schedules, in part because they help improve workload balancing throughout the week.
- Managers and executive leaders see improved outcomes from staff productivity increases, supply management enhancements, facility utilization gains, and service excellence to patients.

LABOR PRODUCTIVITY MANAGEMENT

Demand alignment levers are critical for improving labor management and are often employed in tandem as part of a productivity collaborative team's work. Together, they help leaders achieve a balance of resources with demand while improving workflow by reducing demand variation.

Work and process redesign should precede and drive labor productivity improvements. Organizations must redesign roles and processes to leverage those resources with more available, less costly alternatives. Consequently, roles and processes must continuously evolve to deliver quality care and excellent service at the lowest cost.

For many healthcare leaders, productivity improvement is synonymous with staff reductions. In a common scenario, managers are charged with achieving full-time equivalent staffing targets by a specified date; that mandate frequently arises from a financial urgency to reduce labor costs, necessitating layoffs or reductions in force through attrition. These initiatives often fail to achieve the goal because the fundamental work has not changed and the remaining staff must determine how to get the same workload done with fewer staff members. Without a significant shift in how work is performed (i.e., process improvement), over time, staffing will return to its original levels.

Thus, productivity improvement seeks to minimize labor expense per unit of service (see the following equation) while meeting or exceeding patient service expectations and achieving quality outcomes. The labor cost per unit of service can be lowered by increasing the units of service, reducing the number of hours used, or lowering the average pay rate.

$$\text{Labor \$/Unit of service} = \frac{\text{Labor hours} \times \text{Average pay rate}}{\text{Total unit of service}}$$

A department's actual labor expense per unit of service is a function of many variables. Average pay rates, for example, are a function of the following factors:

- Compensation rates established by the organization
- Protocols for shift differentials, on-call time, and other pay arrangements
- The skill mix of the work group

- The mix of staffing according to pay status (e.g., full time, part time, as needed [pro re nata, or PRN])
- Staff tenure (long-tenured employees are usually at the top of a job class pay range and accrue more paid time off [PTO] than short-tenured staff)
- The amount of overtime, agency, and contracted labor incurred

Healthcare managers must deploy optimal staffing levels that are neither too great nor too little to provide services effectively. From a productivity perspective, key decisions include

- crafting personnel schedules to meet the expected workload requirement,
- determining when additional staffing or overtime is required to cover demand spikes,
- redeploying staff to other locations on the basis of demand shifts,
- deciding when or if a position is added or replaced,
- reassigning roles and responsibilities among staff members, and
- improving processes to increase service effectiveness and efficiency.

How well these decisions are executed determines a department's overall labor productivity performance.

DEMAND MATCHING

As a starting point for resource scheduling, managers must understand the unique demand characteristics of their department or function. Specifically, leaders need clarity on how the volume and mix of demand and workload vary by hour of day, day of week, and season to season. Managers must anticipate when seasonal demand peaks and declines are likely to occur tomorrow, next week, and over the course of the year.

Demand matching is the process of assigning the right number of staff (neither understaffed nor overstaffed) at the right time to perform the required work. Many hospital departments have workload requirements that vary from day to day and can be difficult to predict. Managers must develop flexible staffing plans that are designed for normal workload levels but can flex on the basis of spikes or drops in demand. Effective demand management requires the following:

- A flexible workforce that includes an optimal mix of full-time and part-time staff as well as PRN, on-call, and float staff
- Judicious use of overtime and temporary or agency staffing to fill short-term vacancies or seasonal workload spikes
- Effective role design that balances work across team members and supports cross-coverage of tasks
- The ability to smooth demand workload for schedulable tasks and to manage the balance of deferrable and nondeferrable work
- The ability to anticipate demand in areas where demand is largely unscheduled and to create alternative staff plans when workload is very high or very low

One key healthcare management challenge is planning for and responding to variations in service demand. Demand variation in a hospital setting is shaped by numerous factors inherent in the provision of medical care. For example:

- Inpatient caseload spikes generally occur during the winter months because of the high rate of influenza, pneumonia, and other seasonal maladies.
- Census levels on surgical nursing units are usually high in the early part of the week and decline on Thursdays and

Fridays, reflective of surgical scheduling and the need to discharge patients before the weekend.

- Hospital laboratory workload spikes mid-morning following physician rounding and test ordering.
- Most emergency departments (EDs) see demand peaks in the mid-afternoon and early evening hours.

Hospital-based patient care services have a mix of controllable demand, which is scheduled in advance, and nonscheduled, less predictable demand. A central hospital laboratory, for example, must accommodate a number of components of demand for its services:

- *Testing for inpatients.* Generally predictable, with large demand spikes in the early morning and high volumes occurring on weekdays. Demand continues throughout the day and night.
- *Preadmission testing.* Schedule-driven and largely predictable. Generally, demand occurs during the day shift on weekdays.
- *Outpatient laboratory testing.* Largely schedule-driven, with most demand occurring during the day shift on weekdays.
- *ED patient testing.* Unscheduled and less predictable. Demand occurs throughout the day, with peaks occurring from late afternoon until 9:00 or 10:00 p.m.

Despite these complexities, analyzing hospital service demand can reveal underlying patterns and trends that help leaders anticipate future workload requirements. Leaders need this type of information to develop decision support systems that accurately forecast future demand.

Predictive analytics can provide support in modeling future healthcare staffing and resource requirements. The following case study is an example of how basic predictive analytics is employed to support daily staffing decisions for acute patient care services.

CASE EXAMPLE: PREDICTIVE MODELING FOR ACUTE CARE NURSING

A chief nursing executive of a regional healthcare system was interested in improving the accuracy with which patient care staffing decisions and allocations were determined. The nursing division used a central float pool to support staffing on six nursing units. Nursing managers conducted "bed huddle" meetings three times per day to report on activity and census levels for their units and to estimate their staffing requirements for the next shift.

The bed huddle meetings occurred at 2:30 a.m., 9:30 a.m., and 1:30 p.m. (exhibit 5.1). At each meeting, the nurse managers determined staffing allocations in anticipation of the expected admission and discharge activity over the ensuing hours. Predictions on discharges were made primarily on the basis of information gathered during patient rounding and the experience and intuition of each nurse manager.

Exhibit 5.1: Bed Huddle Meeting Process

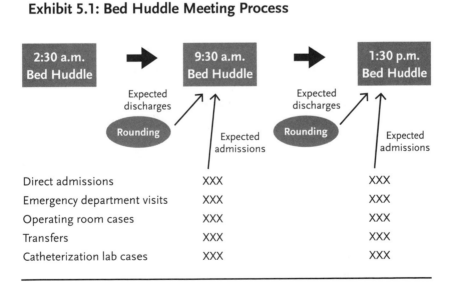

Predicting future census levels was challenging for the latter two huddles, as most of the admission and discharge activity occurred between 10:00 a.m. and 5:00 p.m. The chief nurse wanted to reduce the subjectivity of staffing forecasts by employing a model to forecast expected patient census levels over the next six to eight hours for each patient care unit.

As a starting point, a data analyst evaluated 12 months' worth of daily admission, discharge, and transfer data by hour of day for all nursing units. The information provided insights into the flow of patients between areas and the primary admission sources for each unit. Exhibit 5.2 is a component of the workload analysis for an inpatient orthopedic unit comparing the hourly distribution of transfers in and out on Mondays and Fridays.

As in most surgical units, orthopedic patients are typically admitted early in the week and are discharged by the end of the week. Comparing Mondays to Fridays revealed the following information:

- Most admissions occur on Mondays, creating a spike in activity requiring increased staffing levels.
- Admissions occur over a protracted time interval, with most occurring from 9:00 a.m. to 5:00 p.m.
- On Fridays, staff are primarily occupied with patient discharges. Morning rounds are completed mid-morning, creating a surge in discharges at 10:00 a.m.

The information further revealed the extent of the workload distributions occurring each day of the week and the differences across units.

Next, the analyst built a forecasting model using probability tables by unit of admission from five sources:

- Direct admissions
- Emergency department
- Operating room (OR)
- Interunit transfer
- Catheterization laboratory

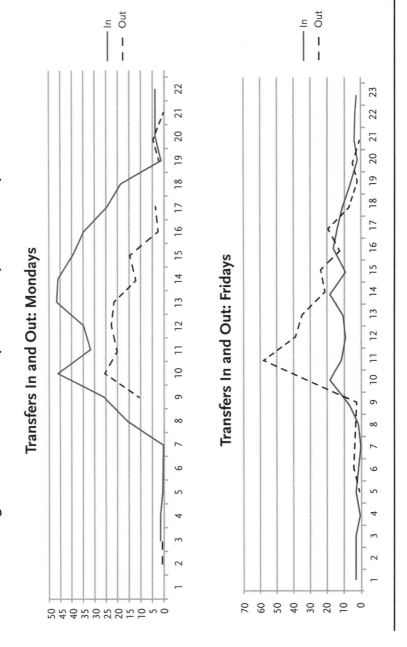

Exhibit 5.2: Average Transfers In and Out by Hour of Day for an Orthopedic Unit

Transfers In and Out: Mondays

Transfers In and Out: Fridays

In
Out

Similar probability tables were developed to predict discharges by hourly increments. By inputting actual total volumes for the five admission sources (actual volumes based on what was occurring at the time of the bed huddle), the model could calculate expected census levels by unit for the next eight hours.

Consequently, the model reduced the subjectivity in determining future census levels on the units. The model dramatically improved the accuracy of the forecast, which improved the assignment of staffing from the float pool.

WORK MEASUREMENT AND ACTIVITY ANALYSIS

Workload drives the need for staffing resources with specific skills required at certain times of the day. When planning a new service, engineering new roles, or developing new team designs, one helpful approach is to construct an activity analysis of the required work. An activity analysis is an inventory of key tasks performed in a department, their frequency, and the time requirements for completion.

Exhibit 5.3 (starting on page 120) is a portion of an activity analysis worksheet for a surgical nursing unit. This template is used to quantify the time spent on patient care tasks to derive a total number of direct hours required per patient day. Task sheets for other departments vary in format and content but serve a similar purpose of quantifying work and skill requirements.

The activity analysis worksheet includes the following components:

- **Task descriptions**. A list of the tasks performed in the department. An acute care nursing unit can have 100 or more specific patient care activities that are performed routinely. Not all departments and functions require this level of specificity.
- **Frequency**. The number of times a task is performed over a defined period. On a nursing unit, some activities are

performed each patient day, whereas other tasks occur intermittently during a patient's stay.

- **Minutes to complete per occurrence**. The average time required to perform the task once.
- **Percentage of patients**. The percentage of cases on the unit for which the activity is performed.
- **Total minutes per stay**. Calculated as Frequency per stay × Minutes to complete per occurrence × Percentage of patients.
- **Minutes per patient day**. Calculated as Total minutes per stay ÷ Average length of stay.
- **Distribution by shift**. The percentage of time by shift for when the activity is typically performed. In this example, the minutes per patient day are distributed across two 12-hour shifts.
- **Deferability**. An indicator of how long a task can be delayed or reassigned to a different time of day. Deferrable tasks are important, but not urgent, activities that can be scheduled and performed at a time that staff are less occupied with nondeferrable work.
- **Minimum skill level**. The lowest skill level that can effectively perform a task. Skill level assignments should not violate any regulatory or licensure requirements.
- **Task constraints**. Consideration of constraints that dictate when or where a task is performed. For example:
  - *Physical constraints*—Does this task require performance in a fixed location? Is the task tied to a specific piece of equipment or technology with limited access? Do any space or facility issues limit the performance of the task?
  - *Time constraints*—Must the task be performed at a specific time of the day? Do off-shift coverage or minimum staffing levels dictate who performs the task?
  - *Process constraints*—Can a task be extracted from other, larger tasks? Will service or patient satisfaction be

affected if everyone who is competent to provide the service does so?

— *Economic and market constraints*—Do retraining costs outweigh the benefits of implementation? What impact will job redesign have on compensation levels? Can we attract staff to the position? Is an adequate supply of this type of worker available in the marketplace?

Exhibit 5.3 is an example of a detailed task analysis in a clinical setting. Activity analysis is equally applicable in nonclinical departments and does not always require the same level of detail. An activity analysis provides a solid foundation of relevant information for aligning staffing with demand. Specifically, the activity analysis provides data to

- determine staff scheduling requirements,
- identify skill mix requirements,
- reschedule deferrable tasks to smooth workload across shifts and days of the week, and
- structure a role and team redesign effort on the basis of the analysis results.

LEVER 4: DEMAND SMOOTHING

Demand smoothing pertains to those interventions and scheduling protocols that seek to balance workload demands and reduce variation during the day and throughout the week. Reducing demand variation enables managers to plan and deploy staffing and other resources with more precision than when variation goes unchecked. The ability to smooth demand variation is highly contingent on the level of control leaders have in scheduling their workload.

Deferrable Work

One method for smoothing workload is to redistribute work to different times of the day or week. For example, an activity analysis includes identifying tasks that are deferrable. Proactively rescheduling deferrable tasks can help departments shift nonurgent work to low-demand days and shifts. Many clinical departments require 24-hour service provision, which can result in underutilized staffing at night and during days of low census. Shifting deferrable tasks to these staff can improve productivity and alleviate some of the workload burden for the peak demand hours.

Demand smoothing would be a straightforward process if all activities were deferrable or healthcare leaders had full control over patient scheduling. Aligning staff and resources with demand is relatively easy when workload is predictable and evenly distributed throughout the day and across the week. However, medical services scheduling is complex and often influenced by factors beyond a manager's direct control. Furthermore, the degree of control over patient scheduling varies with the type of patient and the service provided (exhibit 5.4).

For areas with comprehensive scheduling control, leaders should develop appointment schedules and hours of operation that meet the demands of patients and physicians while distributing the workload as evenly as possible throughout the week. This approach works well in physician offices and most ambulatory services. Conversely, emergency departments are 24-hour operations with few scheduled visits, making demand unpredictable. ED managers must provide sufficient capacity to cover peak demands and have contingency plans in place for those times that workload is significantly higher or lower than expected.

Demand smoothing is critical in areas such as surgical services, where leaders must balance the needs of patients (usually a mix of inpatients, outpatients, and emergency cases) with the scheduling preferences of surgeons. Many hospital surgery programs use block scheduling to preassign ORs and hours to accommodate

Exhibit 5.3: Activity Analysis Worksheet for an Acute Care Unit (partial listing)

7 NORTH—SURGERY

Average length of stay: 4.3

Activity Category	Task Description	Frequency per Patient Day	Frequency per Patient Stay	Minutes per Occurrence	Percentage of Patients	Total Minutes per Stay	Minutes per Patient Day	Estimated Distribution by Shift		Time Distribution by Shift		Deferrable?	Minimum Skill Level
								Day	Night	Day	Night		
A	Coordinating therapy	1.0		4	100.0%	16.2	3.8	80%	20%	3.0	0.8	H	Unlicensed
A	Doppler pulse	3.0		2	80.0%	19.4	4.5	55%	45%	2.0	2.0	H	Unlicensed
A	Circulatory site checks	3.0		1	100.0%	12.1	2.8	80%	20%	2.3	0.6	H	Unlicensed
A	Calf/thigh measurements		1	3	80.0%	2.3	0.5	80%	20%	0.4	0.1	H	Unlicensed
A	Shift assessment	3.0		8	100.0%	97.0	22.6	50%	50%	7.5	11.3	H	Registered nurse
A	Physician consults		2	9	90.0%	16.9	3.9	80%	20%	3.1	0.8	H	Registered nurse
A	Nonphysician consults		6	5	100.0%	28.2	6.6	80%	20%	5.2	1.3	H	Registered nurse
A	Care planning	1.0		6	100.0%	24.3	5.6	75%	25%	4.2	1.4	H	Unlicensed
A	Initial admission/transfer assessment—nurse		1	19	100.0%	18.8	4.4	75%	25%	3.3	1.1	Non	Registered nurse
B	Daily feeding set change	1.0		5	10.0%	2.0	0.5	55%	45%	0.2	0.2	S	Unlicensed
B	Physician rounds	1.0		4	70.0%	11.3	2.6	80%	20%	2.1	0.5	Non	Unlicensed
B	Retrospective physician order check	1.0		2	100.0%	8.1	1.9	80%	20%	1.5	0.4	H	Unlicensed
B	Feeding tube maintenance	3.0		5	10.0%	6.1	1.4	60%	40%	0.6	0.6	Non	Unlicensed

(continued)

(continued from previous page)

Activity Category	Task Description	Frequency per Patient Day	Frequency per Patient Stay	Minutes per Occurrence	Percentage of Patients	Total Minutes per Stay	Minutes per Patient Day	Estimated Distribution by Shift		Time Distribution by Shift		Deferrable?	Minimum Skill Level
								Day	Night	Day	Night		
B	Wound care/dressing—simple	3.0		5	25.0%	15.2	3.5	75%	25%	2.6	0.9	H	Unlicensed
B	Feeding tube insertion		1	9	1.0%	0.1	0.0	80%	20%	0.0	0.0	H	Unlicensed
B	Physician assist—complex process		1	24	10.0%	2.4	0.5	75%	25%	0.4	0.1	Non	Unlicensed
B	Consents/permissions		1	5	10.0%	0.5	0.1	80%	20%	0.1	0.0	S	Unlicensed
B	Scheduling/coordination of physical therapy testing	1.0		5	100.0%	20.2	4.7	80%	20%	3.8	0.9	Non	Registered nurse
B	Physician order sign-off	1.0		3	100.0%	12.1	2.8	80%	20%	2.3	0.6	Non	Registered nurse
B	Physician notification/phone orders	1.0		4	100.0%	16.2	3.8	75%	25%	2.8	0.9	Non	Registered nurse
B	Initiate blood/blood product transfusion		1	19	10.0%	1.9	0.4	75%	25%	0.3	0.1	Non	Registered nurse
B	Central line blood draws		2	9	5.0%	0.9	0.2	75%	25%	0.2	0.1	Non	Registered nurse
B	Emergent situation		1	42	10.0%	4.2	1.0	70%	30%	0.7	0.3	Non	Registered nurse
B	Range of motion	1.0		5	30.0%	6.1	1.4	75%	25%	1.1	0.4	H	Unlicensed
B	Transcription and order entry	1.0		5	100.0%	20.2	4.7	75%	25%	3.5	1.2	Non	Unlicensed
B	Fill water pitchers	2.0		1	100.0%	8.1	1.9	55%	45%	0.8	0.8	H	Unlicensed

Note: H = deferrable to next hour; S = deferrable to next shift; M = deferrable within minutes; non = nondeferrable.

Exhibit 5.4: Degree of Scheduling Control by Clinical Service

Clinical Service	Degree of Patient Scheduling Control	Scheduling Constraints
Physician office care	High control	Patient preferences, physician preferences, office hours, access and capacity
Outpatient rehabilitation and diagnostic services	High control	Patient preferences, staffing and hours of operation, access and capacity
Inpatient surgery	Partial control	Surgeon preferences, anesthesia coverage, room capacity, patient preferences, emergency and add-on cases, staff availability
Inpatient laboratory	Partial control	Unit rounding, emergency and STAT (immediate) testing, scheduled outpatients
Emergency services	Low control	Access and capacity

high-volume surgeons. How well blocks are designed and monitored has a significant impact on workload balancing during the day and throughout the week.

The following case example illustrates the impact of block scheduling on department performance and how improvements can yield improved room utilization and staff productivity.

CASE EXAMPLE: SURGICAL BLOCK SCHEDULING

A new surgical services director was struggling with case scheduling. The organization had block schedules in place for years, but it had not managed the utilization of the blocks with consistency. As dictated by operations policy, surgeons were expected to maintain utilization at 75 percent or higher or risk losing their block assignment. In addition to low block utilization, other issues persisted, including the following:

- Caseload imbalances plagued the surgery department from morning to afternoon, with a significant drop-off in utilization after lunch.
- Most surgeons requested 7:30 a.m. start times; however, urology, general surgery, and surgical oncology surgeons consistently started cases at 8:00 a.m.
- The afternoon blocks for lengthy neurosurgery and cardiovascular procedures frequently bled into the late afternoon, resulting in increased overtime pay for the hospital's surgical staff.
- Few daytime hours went unblocked, creating difficulties in accommodating trauma and other unscheduled cases.

Consequently, the director redesigned the block assignments with the goals of freeing up capacity and improving room and staff utilization. Although the director saw improvement opportunities across the week, she noted that Thursday block schedules were particularly problematic (exhibit 5.5).

In response to findings from the analysis, the director reconfigured the block schedule with the goals of improving block utilization and balancing demand during the day and across the week. Specifically, she

- eliminated several blocks with consistently low utilization;
- moved the afternoon neurosurgery block to the morning to reduce the incidence of late cases;
- adjusted the blocks for urology, general surgery, and surgical oncology to start at 8:00 a.m., enabling the director to stagger staffing and smooth morning demand in the preoperative holding area;

Exhibit 5.5: Surgical Block Scheduling Redesign

Thursday—ORIGINAL BLOCKS

Room #	7:30	8:00	8:30	9:00	9:30	10:00	10:30	11:00	11:30	12:00	12:30	13:00	13:30	14:00	14:30	15:00	15:30
1	Urology block (82%)											Urology block (35%)					
2	General surgery block (85%)											General surgery block (40%)					
3	Cardiovascular block (66%)											Cardiovascular block (45%)					
4	General surgery block (65%)											General surgery block (40%)					
5								Orthopedics block (75%)									
6								Orthopedics block (54%)									
7	Surgical oncology block (65%)																
8	Neurosurgery block (67%)											Neurosurgery block (54%)					
9	Bariatric block (39%)																
10					Orthopedics block (35%)							Ear, nose, and throat block (51%)					
Cysto																	

Indicates assigned block time

Thursday—PROPOSED BLOCKS

Room #	7:30	8:00	8:30	9:00	9:30	10:00	10:30	11:00	11:30	12:00	12:30	13:00	13:30	14:00	14:30	15:00	15:30
1	Urology block (85%)																
2	General surgery block (85%)																
3	Cardiovascular block (68%)																
4	General surgery block (65%)											General surgery block (60%)					
5								Orthopedics block (75%)									
6								Orthopedics block (70%)									
7	Surgical oncology block (65%)																
8	Neurosurgery block (67%)																
9	Neurosurgery block (50%)											Bariatric block (49%)					
10												Ear, nose, and throat block (51%)					
Cysto																	

Note: The percentages represent initial and projected utilization averages.

- moved the bariatric surgery block to the afternoon to free up capacity in the morning; and
- doubled the amount of unblocked time to accommodate unscheduled cases.

The director identified similar improvements for the other weekdays, including a reduction of two staffed rooms on Fridays. She was also able to reconfigure staff scheduling, including the use of more 10-hour-shift employees on Mondays through Thursdays. The director presented her recommendations to the OR leadership committee, which approved the new plan. As a result of these changes, the department achieved the following gains:

- Improved surgeon compliance to block-scheduling protocols
- Increased capacity and flexibility to accommodate unscheduled cases
- Improved OR room utilization during core hours
- Reduced start delays for first cases
- Improved personnel scheduling and productivity

LEVER 5: DEMAND REGROUPING

Grouping work activities with similar labor and resource requirements is generally more efficient than having these same activities dispersed in multiple areas in the organization. This principle holds true in health systems for both clinical and nonclinical operations. The following benefits result from grouping common work:

- Grouping creates a critical mass of like tasks and skill requirements, enabling staff to develop high proficiency levels and improve the quality of the work they perform.
- Regrouping allows for enhanced alignment of staffing and skill mix with the work requirement.

- In some cases, regrouping reduces the need for duplicate equipment and facilities.

Like demand smoothing, demand regrouping seeks to influence the distribution of demand and work requirements to yield predictability and control. The degree of demand regrouping is limited by facility, capacity, patient, and physician constraints.

Patient Regrouping in Acute Care

Demand regrouping is particularly relevant to the organization and management of acute care services (Leander 1996, 87–104). Patients are well served when they are assigned to the unit and care team that is best equipped and experienced to provide for their specific medical needs. For this level of service excellence to occur, hospitals need sufficient bed capacity and designated nursing units that match the organization's mix and volume of inpatient cases. Frequently, hospitals have a misalignment between demand and how units are designated and sized, resulting in similar cases and service lines being spread across multiple units. Often, these units vary in their level of proficiency and staffing models.

Patient regrouping should be an early step in patient care redesign. Effective patient regrouping includes the following steps:

1. Inventory current patient days by nursing unit, diagnosis-related group, and service line to understand where patients currently reside.
2. Identify instances of overutilization of critical care and step-down care resulting in uneven or slow throughput.
3. Build any projected length-of-stay and throughput improvement assumptions into the target design.
4. Identify opportunities to consolidate similar patients into fewer areas. Patient grouping can occur on the basis of several variables, including

a. service line designation,
b. nursing care requirements (e.g., acuity, length of stay, ancillary consumption),
c. physician group involved, and
d. medical versus surgical case designation.
5. Recast census levels under ideal conditions to gauge the potential impact on each unit.
6. Institute processes and systems to support new patient placement strategies.

Exhibit 5.6 is an example of regrouping for patients with cardiopulmonary, cardiovascular surgery, and thoracic surgery diagnoses. This organization regrouped patients to achieve the following goals:

- Reducing critical care usage by moving more patients to the telemetry units
- Grouping more pulmonary medicine cases on the intermediate care unit
- Sending all cardiac surgery patients to the cardiovascular intensive care unit
- Moving medical cardiology patients from intermediate care to the cardiovascular intermediate care unit

The new design provided protocols for assigning patients to the appropriate units and created distinct patient groups on those units. These accomplishments in turn enabled managers to further assign patient cohorts to specific zones in a unit.

Exhibit 5.7 is an example of two patient groupings for a large medical–surgical unit. Group A represents the higher-acuity patients associated with neurosurgery, neurology, and medical cardiology. Group B is composed of less acute medical and surgical cases. The manager designated a portion of the unit to be assigned to both groups, enabling her to institute alternative care team models to address the acuity differences between the two groups.

Exhibit 5.6: Patient Regrouping Example for Cardiovascular and Pulmonary Patients

Average Daily Census Before Regrouping

Service	Critical Care Unit	CV ICU	Telemetry	IMC	CV IMC	Surgical Unit	Total
Cardiology medical	1.8	1.2	5.7	2.5	3.5	0.7	15.4
Pulmonary medical	1.8	1.0	3.9	3.8	2.0	2.6	15.1
Cardiac surgery	1.5	3.5	0.4	0.3	3.2	0.0	8.9
Thoracic surgery	1.7	2.8	0.4	0.7	0.9	0.3	6.8
Vascular intervention	0.6	1.0	0.8	0.8	0.8	1.1	5.1
Cardiology intervention	0.8	1.0	0.8	0.4	1.4	0.0	4.4
Total	**8.2**	**10.5**	**12.0**	**8.5**	**11.8**	**4.7**	**55.7**

Target Average Daily Census After Regrouping

Service	Critical Care Unit	CV ICU	Telemetry	IMC	CV IMC	Surgical Unit	Total
Cardiology medical	1.0	1.7	6.8	0.0	5.9	0.0	15.4
Pulmonary medical	1.5	1.0	3.0	8.1	0.0	1.5	15.1
Cardiac surgery	0.0	5.0	0.4	0.3	3.2	0.0	8.9
Thoracic surgery	1.7	2.8	0.4	0.7	0.9	0.3	6.8
Vascular intervention	0.6	1.0	0.8	0.8	0.8	1.1	5.1
Cardiology intervention	0.8	1.0	0.8	0.4	1.4	0.0	4.4
Total	**5.6**	**12.5**	**12.2**	**10.3**	**12.2**	**2.9**	**55.7**

Note: CV = cardiovascular; ICU = intensive care unit; IMC = intermediate care.

Exhibit 5.7: Patient Grouping Example for a Medical–Surgical Nursing Unit

Patient Group A (12.0)	Patient Group B (17.9)
Neurology and neurosurgery (5.1)	Pulmonary medicine
• Intracranial hemorrhage	Gastroenterology
• Acute ischemic stroke	General medicine
• Transient ischemia	Nephrology
• Traumatic stupor and coma	General surgery
Medical cardiology (5.7)	
• Heart failure and shock	
• Acute myocardial infarction syncope and collapse	
• Cardiac arrhythmia	
Other (1.2)	

Note: Average daily census indicated in parentheses.

Other Examples of Demand Regrouping

The principles of work regrouping are applicable in other clinical and nonclinical areas. Examples include the following:

- *Emergency services*—implementing a "fast track" service for nonurgent, low-acuity patients; providing a chest pain service for cardiac emergency patients
- *Surgical services*—segmenting the OR into zones with designated service lines
- *Patient accounts*—grouping accounts by payer type (e.g., Medicare, Medicaid, commercial insurer) and assigning work teams with specialized knowledge and experience

- *Observation unit*—redeploying observation and other outpatients from multiple inpatient units to a central short-stay unit

Demand regrouping can also occur across entities in a healthcare system. Mature systems consolidate duplicate clinical services to a single site. Under this scenario, patients with specific service needs and diagnoses are directed to a single, central location in a regional system. This strategy pools clinical service demand, creating specialized care sites with focused expertise, sometimes referred to as "focus factories" in other industries (Herzlinger 1997). Like other forms of demand regrouping, clinical rationalization increases economies of scale and builds proficiencies and expertise for staff. Rationalization is explored further in chapter 6.

LEVER 6: ROLE AND TEAM REDESIGN

For many organizations, formal roles and responsibilities (usually delineated in job descriptions) remain static while changes occur in technology, work content, and consumer demand. Performance improvement requires a continuous reevaluation of job design and work team configurations.

Role design is an important and frequently overlooked factor in performance management. Work roles are shaped by

- explicitly assigned tasks and responsibilities;
- informal tasks that are an inherent part of the role;
- skills and formal training and licensure requirements for task performance;
- the number of authorized hours scheduled, the shift worked, and the physical location of the job;
- reporting relationships and management responsibilities; and
- the degree of autonomy inherent in the role.

Demand smoothing and grouping, and the insights gained from activity analyses, help define and quantify workload requirements and the requisite mix and proportion of staffing. Armed with this information, leaders may craft defined roles to perform the work.

Healthcare leaders should approach role redesign with the following collective goals:

- Enhancing service provision for patients and other internal and external customers
- Increasing the flexibility of labor resources to respond to changing workload demand
- Reducing redundant and non-value-added work
- Continuously improving the skills and proficiencies of the workforce
- Developing roles that provide challenge and fulfillment for staff

Effective role design strikes a balance between the production requirements of the organization and staff needs. The organization requires

- a stable supply of skilled labor resources with limited turnover,
- flexibility in human resources to respond to changes in work requirements, and
- committed workers who are motivated and support the organization's mission and values.

For staff, effective role design

- ensures meaningful work that leverages an individual's skills, training, and interests (Manion, Lorimer, and Leander 1996);
- provides opportunities for skill advancement and job promotion;

- provides workers with sufficient compensation commensurate with the skills and work requirements; and
- attracts and retains qualified and motivated staff.

Team Design

Role design for a single position should not occur in isolation but rather should consider how responsibilities and tasks are shared and integrated with other team members. Healthcare system employees rarely work alone. Most services are performed by integrated teams composed of multiple workers with varying skill sets. Numerous examples of work teams are seen in healthcare organizations, such as the following:

- Groups of licensed and unlicensed staff working together on an acute care unit
- Surgery teams composed of surgeons, scrub nurses, and surgical technicians
- Interdisciplinary teams of case managers, social workers, pharmacists, physicians, and caregivers working to transition inpatients to post-acute services
- Groups of account representatives assigned to specific payer categories in the patient accounts area
- Environmental services staff assigned to cover acute care room turnover, terminal cleaning, and other daily facility cleaning
- Home care staff working with case managers, physical therapists, and other providers of post-acute services
- Dyad leadership teams of hospitalists and nurse leaders providing coordinated care on patient care units

Role design forms the basis of team design. Together, they determine how work is distributed within and across multiple skill levels and job categories. To function effectively, work teams should be characterized by the following (Manion, Lorimer, and Leander 1996):

- A relatively small number of people with complementary skills
- A commitment to a shared purpose
- Consistency in membership
- A common working approach and clearly defined roles
- Complementary and overlapping skills
- Mutual accountability

Effective role and team redesign requires a balance of three primary objectives: balanced workload, shared workload, and professional challenge (exhibit 5.8).

Exhibit 5.8: Team Design Objectives

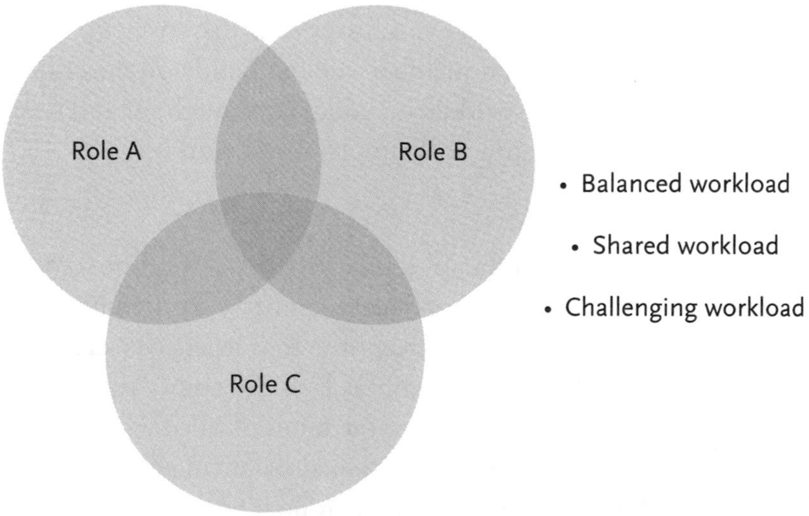

Role A

Role B

Role C

- Balanced workload
- Shared workload
- Challenging workload

Balanced Workload

Effective teams achieve a balance in workload across the team members, so individuals are neither under- nor overutilized. Healthcare leaders should ensure that the work of a department or program is distributed evenly across staff members. Misaligned workload fuels staff dissatisfaction and undermines work performance. Workload imbalances occur when

- roles are poorly designed, or responsibilities are not clearly defined among team members;
- cross-training is insufficient, or a lack of clarity exists regarding shared tasks;
- the staff skill mix and the work requirement are misaligned; and
- individuals lack accountability, motivation, or a sense of teamwork.

Most job responsibilities include a mix of tasks that are time sensitive or urgent and tasks that do not have hard deadlines or immediacy. Effective role design yields a balance of deferrable and nondeferrable responsibilities across each team member. Jobs with a high degree of task urgency can foster staff dissatisfaction and burnout. In such cases, staff members are frequently on the critical path of a team's primary workflow, reducing throughput and team productivity and preventing the completion of work.

Shared Workload

A balanced workload is difficult to achieve when few of the responsibilities and tasks overlap among team members. Workgroups with minimal shared workload are susceptible to bottlenecks and poor customer service when team members lack the ability to respond quickly to patient requests. Cross-trained, multiskilled workers help maintain staffing flexibility and workload balancing. The benefits of multiskilled work teams include the following:

- *Reduced downtime.* Multiskilled teams can reduce the downtime frequently associated with narrowly focused role designs, as more team members are qualified to provide a service.
- *Parallel task processing.* Multiskilled workers integrate new responsibilities into their current workflow in a manner that simplifies processes and reduces duplicate and non-value-added work.
- *Improved service responsiveness.* Multiskilled workers can respond quickly to patients' and other customers' needs by reducing unnecessary handoffs to other associates.
- *Improved productivity.* Multiskilled staff increase the flexibility of labor resources for demand matching and enable organizations to achieve higher levels of productivity.

Professional Challenge

Effective job design produces roles that are rewarding and meaningful for incumbents and leverages their skills, training, and abilities. A majority (typically 50 to 70 percent) of professional roles should be composed of tasks requiring their specific license, training, and skills. Higher percentages can limit team flexibility and cross-coverage, and therefore should be avoided.

When possible, care team design should support the continuity of caregivers for individual patients across the course of their stay. Caregiver continuity can result in improved patient and staff satisfaction while enhancing care management. Furthermore, continuity helps build strong teamwork among staff who have experience working together.

Staff members should receive training and be proficient in those tasks that are shared within and across multiple skill levels. The following factors should be considered when designing roles, cross-training, and workload balancing:

- *Licensure constraints.* Cross-training should not violate licensure requirements and regulations that restrict task performance. For example, certain clinical tasks must be performed by registered nurses (RNs), pharmacists, physical therapists, physicians, or other professionals as mandated by law and regulations. Violating these requirements exposes the organization to risks related to loss of accreditation, patient safety, and revenue generation.
- *Concentrated consumption.* Cross-training should focus on tasks performed with high frequency and constitute a sizable amount of total staff time and effort.
- *Competency maintenance.* Cross-trained staff must be able to perform a task with enough frequency to maintain proficiency. The minimum frequency required depends on the task's complexity. The cross-training plan for each task should identify the minimum frequencies of performance required to build an individual's competency and maintain ongoing proficiency.

Role clarity is a significant factor in a team's performance. The following case is an example of how leaders employed principles of team design in an emergency services department.

CASE EXAMPLE: ROLE DESIGN IN AN EMERGENCY DEPARTMENT

A mid-sized suburban community hospital sought to improve the throughput of and waiting time for patients in the ED. At the time, the department had an average length of stay of 4.2 hours, with significantly longer times for patients waiting to be admitted. The leadership team chartered five multidisciplinary collaborative teams to address different dimensions of the ED throughput process.

One team was responsible for improving the existing care team model to increase service to patients. Members of the collaborative team identified lack of role clarity between RNs, paramedics, and patient care technicians as a major operational challenge in the department. The lack of clarity among roles and inconsistent skills among staff resulted in

- ambiguity about expectations of individual team members,
- workload imbalances among individuals and across skill levels and care teams,
- unnecessary work handoffs and missed assignments, and
- general staff dissatisfaction.

Lacking clarity about work responsibilities, the caregivers defaulted to an inflexible, functional assignment of tasks with little work sharing between the RNs and other caregivers. The team conceded that this practice contributed to delays in care that increased the average length of stay for patients and reduced patient satisfaction. The team concluded that the redesigned care model should include delineation of specific nondeferrable care tasks that should be performed by any available caregiver.

As a starting point, the team leader facilitated a brainstorming session with the team to list patient care tasks performed by nurses and other team members. The team identified more than 60 separate patient care tasks performed routinely in the department (exhibit 5.9). From this list, the team identified ten key tasks to designate as shared responsibilities among licensed and nonlicensed staff. These tasks were chosen because they are

- time sensitive and nondeferrable,
- performed frequently,
- time consuming relative to other ED tasks,
- able to be performed in combination with other tasks, and
- not restricted by licensure requirements,

These recommendations were reviewed and approved by the hospital's executive. Select team members were involved in the

Exhibit 5.9: Task Assignments in an Emergency Department

Registered Nurse		Shared Tasks	Paramedic/Technician	
Assessment—initial and ongoing	Blood product verification	Arterial line setup	Evaluation of pain level	Discontinuation of IV site
Advanced triage protocols—ordering	External jugular monitoring	Chest tube setup	Evaluation of changes in patient status	Nasogastric tube insertion
Oral medication administration	Arterial blood gas monitoring	Vigileo setup (central line)	Initial triage/patient routing	Foley catheter insertion and monitoring
Intravenous (IV), intramuscular, or subcutaneous medication administration	Continuous bladder irrigation	Cervical spine precautions	Advanced triage protocols (initiate)	Straight catheter urine collection
Medication effect monitoring	Ear irrigation	Dressing changes	Vital sign documentation and monitoring	Venipuncture
Patient phone inquiry	Nasopharyngeal or throat swabbing/respiratory syncytial virus washing	Delivery of specimens	Visual acuity testing	Cardiac monitoring/posting strips
Code blue coordination	Eye flushing	Patient feeding	Urine collection	X-ray order entry
Arterial line monitoring	Nasogastric tube lavage	Patient ambulation	Stool collection	12-lead electrocardiogram testing
Chest tube monitoring	Implanted tube access	Provision of basic comfort measures (e.g., blankets)	Oxygen therapy	Orthopedic equipment application

(continued)

(continued from previous page)

Exhibit 5.9: Task Assignments in an Emergency Department

Registered Nurse		Shared Tasks	Paramedic/Technician	
Vigileo monitoring	Peripherally inserted central catheter line monitoring	Provision of family support	Orthostatics	Crutch use training
Pelvic monitoring	Critical patient transport coordination		Hold for lumbar puncture	Splint application
Cardiac pacing	Equipment checks		Hold for lacerations (papoose)	Suture/staple removal
Defibrillation	Crash cart checks		Glucose monitoring	External warming therapies
Discharge teaching	Transport tracking		IV initiation	Assistance with patient elimination/enema administration
			IV maintenance and monitoring	Seizure precautions
			Discontinuation of IV fluids	Patient restraint application
				Hard restraint use documentation

implementation process, which included communication and training for all caregivers. The ten tasks were communicated to staff as activities to be performed by "any available team member." The clarity of and focus on specific tasks enabled team members to hold each other accountable for service to patients.

Task sharing proved to be an important factor in improving the department's throughput by 35 percent. Additionally, patient satisfaction scores improved after implementing the role changes.

Patient Care Team Design

Inpatient nurse staffing can represent one third or more of a hospital's workforce. Health systems require sound processes and systems for ensuring effective patient care team design and performance. Team design must incorporate the dimensions of workload balance, shared work, and professional challenge.

Exhibit 5.10 depicts an approach for developing a team design in acute care nursing. While this example focuses on team design for nursing units, similar processes can be applied to other clinical and nonclinical areas in a health system. They include the following:

- **Current staffing models**. Team design begins with an evaluation of the current team model and the licensure and regulatory constraints that set parameters on how work is performed. This assessment should reveal areas where staffing is working well and where productivity and service issues exist. External benchmarking can be useful to understand how other organizations staff and manage similar patient populations and to set targeted staff hours per patient day.
- **Activity analysis**. As part of assessing current practices, it is useful to inventory those tasks and activities routinely performed in a department or work area. The task inventory is used to construct an activity analysis template.

Exhibit 5.10: Patient Care Team Design Process

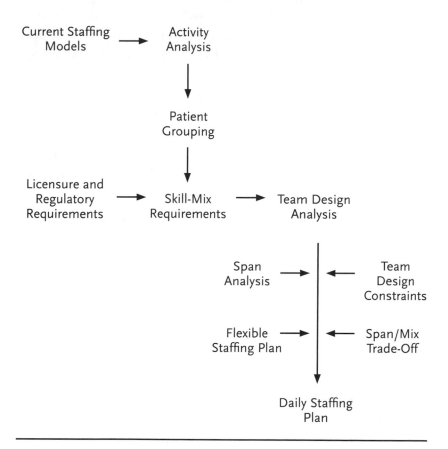

The activity analysis reflects the current staffing models and work assignments, and it reveals the minimum required skill mix (see exhibit 5.3). The results of the activity analysis provide the analytic foundation for deriving an optimal team design.

- **Patient grouping**. Team design should be based on groupings and unit locations for the types of patients served. Any changes to current patient assignments should be factored into the team redesign.

- **Span/mix trade-off**. A collaborative team can test different options by varying the number and mix of caregivers (licensed and nonlicensed) as well as the span of patients-to-caregiver ratios. The team span varies with the size and skill mix of the team as well as patient acuity and the time of day (shift).

  Numerous examples can be found of skill mix decisions that must be made when designing care teams for the following areas:
  - *Nursing*. Team design for acute care units to determine the optimal mix of licensed to nonlicensed staff on the basis of the patient population
  - *Surgery*. Staffing mix and team design for scrub nurses, technicians, and support staff
  - *Physician practices*. Determination of the optimal physician-to–mid-level practitioner mix and nurse-to–medical assistant mix
  - *Pharmacy*. Determination of the optimal pharmacist-to–pharmacy technician mix
  - *Rehabilitative services*. Determination of the optimal therapist-to–therapy technician mix

- **Team design constraints**. Limitations are introduced to further validate optional team designs. Constraints may include facility issues (e.g., unit layout, number of beds, types and sizes of rooms, availability of monitoring technology), patient population issues (e.g., acuity, number, and mix of patients), proximity to equipment and ancillary services, and other issues that affect staffing requirements.

- **Flexible staffing plan**. From the core design model developed during this process, the design team can create daily staffing plans on the basis of varying patient census and acuity levels. Typically, a nursing unit has in place a staffing matrix that determines when and what type of staff is added according to patient census.

The optimal model is cost-effective (minimizes average labor cost per patient day) and achieves the goals of workload balance, shared workload, and professional challenge. Exhibit 5.11 is an example of a patient care staffing matrix for an orthopedic surgery unit with an average daily census of 19 that is staffed using 12-hour shifts. The overall targeted hours per patient day is 9.30, inclusive of management and supervisory positions. If a unit has multiple patient groupings, a similar matrix can be developed for each group.

Team Design Implementation

Team redesign changes the daily work for associates and alters how staff should interact. It can also produce a shift in the culture of a team or program. For these reasons, healthcare leaders must provide the appropriate level of implementation planning and support.

Effective job redesign implementation requires the following components:

- *Investment in training and development.* Staff must have adequate training on newly assigned tasks and responsibilities. Furthermore, task performance must occur with enough frequency to ensure sufficient proficiency.
- *Team building.* Team redesign requires staff to learn new habits and break old ones regarding staff interactions and teamwork among individuals with different skill levels and from different disciplines. Early in implementation, leaders should seek opportunities to build and reinforce new behaviors through team-building events and exercises. Successful team building retains the existing cultural dimensions and practices that work well while adopting required changes to support the new design.
- *New job descriptions, policies, and procedures.* Leaders should update documentation to support the new roles and processes. Updated formal job descriptions and

Exhibit 5.11: Orthopedic Unit Staffing Grid

Unit: Orthopedics   Target Total Hours per Patient: 9.46

Census	Manager	Days CS/TL	RN	LPN	CNA	WC	Nights CS/TL	RN	LPN	CNA	WC	Days Patient-to-Nurse Ratio	Nights Patient-to-Nurse Ratio	Direct Care Hours	Direct Hours per Patient	Total Hours per Patient	Patient-to-CNA Ratio Day Shift	Night Shift
31	0.7	1	6	2	3	1	1	4	2	2	0	3.9	5.2	228	7.35	8.79	10.3	15.5
30	0.7	1	6	2	3	1	1	4	2	2	0	3.8	5.0	228	7.60	9.09	10.0	15.0
29	0.7	1	5	2	3	1	1	4	1	2	0	4.1	5.8	204	7.03	8.57	9.7	14.5
28	0.7	1	5	2	3	1	1	4	1	2	0	4.0	5.6	204	7.29	8.88	9.3	14.0
27	0.7	1	5	2	3	1	1	4	1	2	0	3.9	5.4	204	7.56	9.21	9.0	13.5
26	0.7	1	5	2	3	1	1	4	1	2	0	3.7	5.2	204	7.85	9.56	8.7	13.0
25	0.7	1	4	2	3	1	1	4	1	2	0	4.2	5.0	192	7.68	9.47	8.3	12.5
24	0.7	1	4	2	3	1	1	3	1	2	0	4.0	6.0	180	7.50	9.36	8.0	12.0
23	0.7	1	4	2	2	1	1	3	1	2	0	3.8	5.8	168	7.30	9.25	11.5	11.5
22	0.7	1	4	2	2	1	1	3	1	2	0	3.7	5.5	168	7.64	9.67	11.0	11.0
21	0.7	1	4	1	1	1	1	3	1	2	0	4.2	5.3	144	6.86	8.98	21.0	10.5
20	0.7	1	4	1	1	1	1	3	1	2	0	4.0	5.0	144	7.20	9.43	20.0	10.0
19	0.7	1	4	1	1	1	1	3	1	1	0	3.8	4.8	132	6.95	9.30	19.0	19.0
18	0.7	1	4	1	1	1	1	2	1	1	0	3.6	6.0	120	6.67	9.15	18.0	18.0
17	0.7	1	3	1	1	1	1	2	1	1	0	4.3	5.7	108	6.35	8.98	17.0	17.0

(continued)

(continued from previous page)

Exhibit 5.11: Orthopedic Unit Staffing Grid

Unit: Orthopedics **Target Total Hours per Patient: 9.46**

Census	Manager	Days CS/TL	Days RN	Days LPN	Days CNA	Days WC	Nights CS/TL	Nights RN	Nights LPN	Nights CNA	Nights WC	Days Patient-to-Nurse Ratio	Nights Patient-to-Nurse Ratio	Direct Care Hours	Direct Hours per Patient	Total Hours per Patient	Patient-to-CNA Ratio Day Shift	Patient-to-CNA Ratio Night Shift
16	0.7	1	3	1	1	1	1	2	1	0	0	4.0	5.3	96	6.00	8.79	16.0	
15	0.7	1	3	1	1	1	1	2	1	0	0	3.8	5.0	96	6.40	9.38	15.0	
14	0.7	1	3	1	1	1	0	2	1	0	0	3.5	4.7	96	6.86	9.19	14.0	
13	0.7	1	3	1	1	0	0	2	1	0	0	3.3	4.3	96	7.38	8.97	13.0	
12	0.7	1	2	1	1	0	0	2	1	0	0	4.0	4.0	84	7.00	8.72	12.0	
11	0.7	1	2	1	0	0	0	2	1	0	0	3.7	3.7	72	6.55	8.42		
10	0.7	1	2	1	0	0	0	2	1	0	0	3.3	3.3	72	7.20	9.26		
9	0.7	0	2	1	0	0	0	2	1	0	0	3.0	3.0	72	8.00	8.96		
8	0.7	0	2	0	0	0	0	2	0	0	0	4.0	4.0	48	6.00	7.08		
7	0.7	0	2	0	0	0	0	2	0	0	0	3.5	3.5	48	6.86	8.09		
6	0.7	0	2	0	0	0	0	2	0	0	0	3.0	3.0	48	8.00	9.44		
						Hours per shift: 12					Hours per shift: 12							

Note: Shaded census range represents 80% of the days in the year the census will fall in this range. CNA = certified nurse assistant; CS = clinical specialist; LPN = licensed practical nurse; RN = registered nurse; TL = team leader; WC = ward clerk.

policies should clearly convey the new intended design and provide guidance for managers and staff.

- *Potential realignment of the compensation system.* In some situations, new roles require consideration of a new compensation strategy. Some staff may inherit roles that require a higher skill level and may justify a higher compensation level. Other changing roles may warrant compensation that includes an incentive component. Leaders should understand how redesigned roles affect pay expectations and how a redesigned compensation strategy could provide support to the new design.

- *Recruitment, orientation, and retention strategies.* New team and role design usually requires changes in the recruitment and orientation systems. As new staff join a team or department, leaders need orientation processes in place that preserve the integrity of the redesigned roles and communicate expectations regarding teamwork and staff collaboration.

- *Communication to the rest of the organization.* Team and role redesign can affect other departments and staff in the organization. Leaders must communicate major design changes taking place in their department to the rest of the organization. From the start, leaders should clearly articulate the purposes for change, thereby laying a strong foundation for redesign.

LEVER 7: DYNAMIC STAFFING

The previous six improvement levers enable leaders to

- streamline core processes and facilities to improve service and reduce non-value-added work,
- influence controllable demand through scheduling and regrouping to minimize variation and balance workload, and

- design roles and team models to meet demand with the optimal skill mix.

Next, leaders must develop and execute plans for scheduling and deploying resources in an optimal manner. Health system demand can be highly volatile or unpredictable, making it difficult to optimize staffing at the department level. Matching staffing and physical capacity to changing workload is a daily challenge for department and program leaders. Managers routinely adjust staffing and other resources to accommodate daily demand in their areas of responsibility.

Dynamic staffing is the collective practices and techniques managers employ to plan and schedule staffing and other resources. Effective demand matching ensures that the right skills and resources are available at the right time for patients, physicians, and other internal and external customers.

Strategies that feature dynamic staffing can apply to a single hospital or encompass resource allocation across multiple hospitals and business units. The most common dynamic staffing strategies include the following:

- Using flexible staffing to meet variable workload requirements
- Instituting centralized float pools
- Floating staff from other departments
- Implementing conditional staffing plans in departments with unpredictable workload
- Designing organization-wide seasonal staffing plans

Performance improvement initiatives often address issues of suboptimal staffing and scheduling practices. The many complexities pertaining to staff scheduling in a health system can impede productivity and service performance. Enhancing staff schedules and improving labor alignment can often accelerate performance improvement and reduce labor expenses.

Core Staffing

Dynamic staffing strategies apply predominantly to those programs and services with demand that varies directly or indirectly with patient workload. For these areas, managers should initially establish core staffing levels and then design flexing strategies to increase or decrease staffing as workload changes.

As a starting point, this type of operational area, known as a variable department, should define core staffing levels that accommodate the normal demand range (generally 75–85 percent of the days a program provides service). Ideally, the schedule should include a mix of full-time and part-time staffing to enable coverage of peak workload that occurs at points during the day and for peak days during the week. Managers should determine workload thresholds when staffing is added to or removed from core staffing.

In exhibit 5.12, volumes for a physical therapy department are shown as ranges of production that occur during the year. For 75 percent of the days, the production ranges between 251 and 400 procedures. With this information, a manager can schedule a core staff of members who are able to perform up to 400 procedures per day. For days exceeding this range, the manager must have a surge plan in place to accommodate the additional workload. For days below 251, the manager must proactively reduce staffing from the core.

Flexing Staff Upward

Both of the dynamics involved in flexing staff resources—surging capacity and scaling it back—have their own challenges and necessary approaches. When a surge in demand occurs, a leader can use the options discussed next.

Pro re Nata
PRN staffing is applicable to most areas of a health system. PRN staff are used on an as-needed basis and typically do not receive benefits

Exhibit 5.12: Core and Noncore Staffing

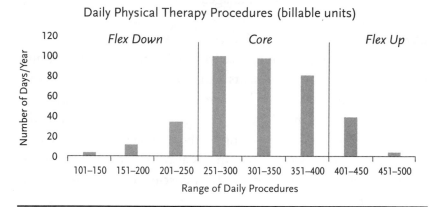

Daily Physical Therapy Procedures (billable units)

or a guaranteed number of hours. PRN staffing provides coverage when core staff are on PTO or to accommodate seasonal demand spikes. A few critical issues must be noted regarding PRN staffing:

- The organization takes on the same risks and responsibilities for the work of PRN staff as with payroll staff. PRN staff must be properly trained and have proficiency in the work they perform.
- Without sufficient oversight, PRN staffing may continue to be used beyond its need. PRN should be an alternative method of filling budgeted, authorized hours, not as an exception to the budget.
- Wage and hour laws place limits on how many hours an individual is paid for PRN-status work.

Agency Staffing
Healthcare systems use agency staffing to fill critical open positions and provide capacity during periods of high, seasonal demand. Agency staffing is most commonly employed in nursing services but can be used for physical therapy and other areas where recruiting is

difficult. Agency staffing is an expensive option for most organizations and should be closely managed.

Overtime

Overtime usage is a common occurrence in many areas of a health system, and it usually represents 2 to 4 percent of a hospital's total paid hours. Clinical areas such as surgery, the cardiac catheterization laboratory, medical imaging, and emergency services are among the highest users of overtime, owing to the emergent and unpredictable nature of their work. Overtime is also a short-term option for filling vacant positions and can be a cost-effective alternative to agency staffing.

Some structured overtime can be cost-effective for departments requiring routine after-hours and weekend coverage. Without sufficient oversight, managers may use overtime excessively. Leaders should budget and manage overtime like any other component of the operating budget.

On-Call Staffing

On-call staffing is appropriate for after-hours coverage of services that are required for clinical emergencies. On-call staffing is found in surgery, medical imaging, cardiac catheterization, and other areas. Call teams usually are paid an hourly rate plus a premium "call back" rate (usually with a minimum time requirement) when called in for a case.

The cost-effectiveness of a call team depends on the actual utilization of the team (i.e., how frequently it is called in). At the point where the sum of on-call and call-back time exceeds regular staffing, the more advantageous option may be to add positions to core staffing.

Central Float Pools

Healthcare organizations frequently employ staffing pools for some clinical service areas. Central staffing pools are useful in a single organization as well as across multiple system entities to provide daily coverage for staffing gaps and to enable surge capacity when demand is high. The most common application of float pools in healthcare is for acute care nurse staffing. Many hospitals employ nursing float pools to allocate daily staffing resources across multiple inpatient units.

A number of factors determine the effectiveness of a nursing float pool:

- *Scale*. Float pools require a minimum scale in the number of units supported and the number of patients served. A single hospital with fewer than 300 beds, for example, may not benefit from a float pool to the same degree that a large organization or a hospital that is part of a larger regional system does.
- *Participation*. Float pools provide an option for individuals seeking flexibility in their hours and pay. The number of individuals must be sufficient to populate the pool with the collective skills to support the hospital's numerous services. Participation levels depend on the supply of nurses and other market factors. The organization must offer compensation levels, and possibly benefits, that attract and retain qualified staff.
- *Predictability*. Float personnel, like other individuals, require some degree of predictability in scheduled hours and location. For example, most caregivers prefer to work in a limited number of areas or departments. To maintain satisfaction and participation levels, staff members should expect to receive a routine number of weekly hours.
- *Proficiency*. For float pools to perform effectively, individuals in the pool must have sufficient hours to retain them and maintain their skills and proficiencies. The number of service areas in which most individuals can perform effectively is limited. For example, finding

an RN who is equally proficient in critical and noncritical care is uncommon. Float pools should be supported by an inventory of existing skills, experience, and licensure for all float personnel to ensure the right staff are assigned to the right clinical area.

Floating Staff

As an alternative to float pools, small organizations can achieve labor flexing by floating staff to other units and departments on the basis of patient and case volumes. To work effectively, float plans must address some of the same proficiency and predictability issues found with central float pools. They also require uniformity in standards of care, staff development, and performance expectations.

Float staffing is applicable to nonclinical as well as clinical staff. For example, a portion of an organization's environmental services staff can be cross-trained to transport patients or serve as patient sitters. These staff may be deployed to different functions as needed to fill vacant positions or meet unexpectedly high demand.

Some regional multihospital systems implement float staffing to coordinate and deploy resources for numerous skilled and technical roles. Cross-entity floating can be applied to pharmacy, surgical nursing, imaging technology, laboratory, physical and occupational therapy, and other professions.

Regional float staffing is limited by geographic distance and location. Most individuals prefer to work at locations in proximity to their home. A regional system with hospitals nearby generally has more success with system floating than geographically dispersed systems have.

Conditional Staffing Plans

Some departments may institute plans that adjust staffing, processes, and roles during a shift to meet unanticipated workload. Conditional staffing plans are useful for instances when throughput must be expedited. Some EDs, for example, institute conditional staffing plans in accordance with the number of patients in the department or when waiting times are excessive. Similar plans can be used to accelerate bed turnover on inpatient units or expedite transfers from the ICU to free up capacity for ED admissions.

Effective conditional staffing plans

- define the conditions under which the department shifts from its core staffing plan to the contingency plan,
- specify the roles of each staff member under each scenario of the contingency plan,
- delineate where staff are physically redeployed when the plan is activated, and
- define the conditions when the department reverts to the core staffing plan.

Flexing Staff Downward

Managers should also have contingency plans for reducing staff when workload is low. Options for flexing staff downward include the following:

- Reduce PRN staffing.
- Encourage use of PTO.
- Send staff home early on slow days.
- Temporarily assign staff to a different department.

These strategies are effective in instances when the workload downturn is expected to be temporary. If reduced workload is expected to be permanent, managers must consider permanent staffing reductions and work redesign to rebalance staffing with the reduced workload.

Seasonal Staffing Plans

Many health systems experience considerable seasonal workload peaks and valleys during the year. Such organizations may institute a seasonal staffing plan for each department. The plan defines target staffing levels for different periods in the year, including peak staffing during busy months and reduced staffing during the off-season.

Frequently, seasonal plans include flexible targets for administrative and support areas with fixed staffing. In the following case study, a hospital system with high seasonality developed seasonal staffing plans for all departments, including fixed administrative areas.

CASE EXAMPLE: SEASONAL STAFFING PLAN

A regional healthcare system implemented a productivity monitoring system to manage staffing in all areas of the organization. For fixed departments, the organization instituted variable standards on the basis of budgeted productive hours per adjusted patient day (patient days adjusted for outpatient activity).

Managers in these areas found flex staffing challenging, particularly in the off-season, resulting in significant budget overages. For this reason, the executive team designed and implemented a seasonal staffing plan for all fixed departments. The goal of the plan was to provide guidelines and protocols for aligning staffing levels with predictable seasonal changes in patient volumes.

From an analysis of adjusted patient days data, leaders identified three levels of patient volumes that occur at predictable points in the year (exhibit 5.13). From this information, the organization developed cost center–specific staffing targets for each period (defined as plans A, B, and C). Additionally, the leaders defined actions to occur during each period to manage hiring and attrition, the use of flex staffing, and the scheduling of time off.

Exhibit 5.13: Seasonal Staffing Plan

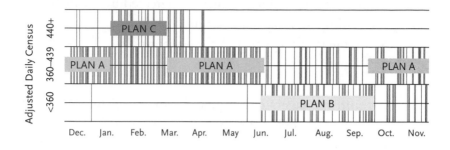

- *Plan A—core staffing* (adjusted patient day [APD] range 360–440):
  - Active 60 percent of the time (31 weeks), primarily March through May and October through December (excluding holidays)
  - Assumes normal use of PTO
  - Vacant positions recruited for and filled beginning in September and continuing through April
- *Plan B—reduced staffing* (APD 360 or fewer):
  - Active 25 percent of the time (13 weeks), primarily June through September and holidays
  - Represents a reduction in productive hours of 5 to 11 percent
  - Assumes accelerated use of PTO
  - Eliminates PRN and overtime staffing
  - Reduces staff hours to eight hours per week per FTE
  - Hold placed on recruitment for and filling of open positions from May through August
- *Plan C—augmented staffing* (APD 440 or greater):
  - Active 15 percent of the time (eight weeks), primarily January through February (excluding holidays)

- Represents up to a 20 percent increase in productive hours for select departments
- Assumes restricted use of PTO
- For select fixed departments, increased use of PRN staffing and limited overtime
- Same staffing as plan A for remaining fixed departments

As a result, managers could plan for expected increases and decreases in workload. The new guidelines improved decisions on when to initiate staff hiring and when to leave positions open during the off-season.

CHAPTER 6

Leveraging the System

NUMEROUS REASONS CAN explain why hospital systems join forces and consolidate under a single regional system. Large delivery systems have great market clout with payers and higher brand recognition with patients. In addition, increasing scale enables large systems to rationalize, or reduce redundancies related to, fixed operating expenses and provide care at lower costs.

High-performing regional health systems share common attributes that differ from other organizations:

- They maintain a strong, recognized brand that is uniformly known across the markets they serve.
- Patients can expect high-quality, consistent clinical care and outcomes across these systems.
- Patients tend to experience high-performing customer service from associates throughout these systems.
- Patients can expect timely access and seamless coordination between system entities.
- The collective scale of these systems enables their entities to operate more efficiently than they can on their own.
- Regionalization decisions are made in a manner that improves large systems' ability to compete in the marketplace and to meet patient requirements.

Building these competencies takes time. System-level operational improvement typically evolves over a span of years along a continuum of increasing strategic and operational integration. Most systems initially focus on consolidating market share and improving contracting terms with payers. A large system affiliation enhances a hospital's ability to improve its negotiation leverage and achieve favorable pricing for patient care services.

As systems form, performance and cost improvements frequently remain at the entity level. In fact, overall operating performance during this time can dip as a result of diluted management attention and other factors associated with a merger. Early in a system's formation, a common strategy is to centralize some administrative and support functions. Supply chain, revenue cycle, human resources, and other administrative services are often the first areas to consolidate, helping build initial continuity and standardization across the system.

Disruptive change, such as clinical program consolidation, can occur years after systems form. The speed at which leaders pursue cost savings and operational consolidation is a function of financial urgency, the organization's operating structure, its ability to assimilate diverse cultures, and many other factors.

The levers presented to this point in the book apply predominantly to the process or cross-functional levels in departments and single entities. The three improvement levers discussed in this section represent areas of operational benefit that accrue across entities in healthcare systems. These levers are the following:

- *Management restructuring*—altering the management structure as enabled by rationalizing leadership across multiple departments or sites
- *System rationalization*—leveraging the scale of large systems to reduce redundant programs and spread fixed costs, particularly through centralization
- *Service redeployment*—reallocating staffing and other resources to improve services and reduce expenses

The operating and cost improvements achievable through these levers can be significant. Increasingly, healthcare systems need to leverage system-level opportunities to accelerate performance and achieve increased levels of efficiency and effectiveness.

LEVER 8: MANAGEMENT RESTRUCTURING

The continuing consolidation of hospitals into large regional systems creates opportunities for organizations to leverage and streamline management resources across multiple entities. Management restructuring should occur early in the development of a healthcare system because, in addition to reducing labor expense, a consolidated leadership team is best positioned to drive postmerger program and operational consolidation.

Management positions, including supervisors, managers, directors, and executive staff, typically account for 12 to 18 percent of a healthcare organization's total payroll expenses. Historically, hospitals employed large numbers of leaders and operated with many management layers. Today, directors and mid-level hospital managers commonly have numerous direct reports and administrative responsibilities over multiple departments and programs.

Performance improvement (PI) initiatives often include evaluating leadership positions and structure with the goal of reducing management layers and redundancies. Leadership roles represent most of the highly compensated positions in organizations. For this reason, many healthcare organizations focus on reducing management resources to generate short-term savings while minimizing the total number of individuals affected by workforce reductions.

Management restructuring initiatives are generally directed by collaborative teams composed of system executive leaders, including site CEOs; chief operating officers; and regional-level leaders, including the senior human resources executive. The output of these teams is a new organizational structure that is designed for increased efficiency and supportive of the system's strategic and operational objectives.

Management restructuring should begin with a span-of-control analysis (exhibit 6.1), which inventories all management positions and records the number of direct reports for each leader. Equipped with an inventory of leadership positions across the system, a team can review individual span-of-control data and identify opportunities on a function-by-function basis to streamline leadership resources.

The span-of-control analysis process helps organizations

- clarify reporting relationships,
- quantify organizational span and hierarchy,
- highlight departmental fragmentation,
- reveal excessive management layers, and
- identify those that operate with too many or too few leaders.

Span-of-control analysis should start at the executive level and move downward. Span requirements and the ratio of managers to supervisors vary by functional area. Any redesign to the current management structure should account for these differences. Actual leadership mix ratios should be compared to industry benchmarks to determine areas that are over- or underresourced with management positions. This determination should be made for all levels of management staffing, typically defined according to the following categories:

- Level 1—CEO
- Level 2—vice president and senior vice president
- Level 3—department and program director
- Level 4—manager and assistant director
- Level 5—supervisor and coordinator

Exhibit 6.1: Management Span-of-Control Analysis (partial list)

Functional Category	Supervisor Level					Manager/Director Level				
	Current FTEs	Total Direct Reports	Staff-to-Supervisor Ratio	Supvisor Target Ratio	Supervisors Over/Under	Current FTEs	Total Direct Reports	Staff-to-Manager Ratio	Manager Target Ratio	Managers Over/Under
Accounting/business office	6.0	40.0	6.7	10.1	2.0	3.0	14.0	4.7	3.6	−0.9
Nutrition services	6.0	69.0	11.5	20.5	2.6	4.0	22.0	5.5	6.9	0.8
Patient care—ancillary	15.0	138.0	9.2	25.0	9.5	6.0	43.5	7.3	7.2	0.0
Patient care—general nursing	22.0	530.3	24.1	30.0	4.3	8.0	55.0	6.9	5.4	−2.2
Patient care—ambulatory/therapy	12.0	125.0	10.4	15.0	3.7	6.0	35.0	5.8	6.9	0.9
Home health	5.0	105.4	21.1	15.0	−2.0	2.0	15.0	7.5	5.5	−0.7

Note: FTE = full-time equivalent.

Regional Management Restructuring

The work of the management restructuring collaborative team is critical to the future of an organization. The redesigned leadership structure will have considerable influence on how the system is governed, who provides leadership, and how services are provided going forward. Redesign must account for a system's unique characteristics, including the number, size, and geographic dispersion of hospitals and other entities, as well as market considerations that dictate where services should be located.

The collaborative team should review each program or function and determine the appropriate regional leadership structure. The function and nature of the work performed determine how leadership resources should be assigned to a service. Some administrative and support services lend themselves to a centralized management model, whereas other services must be managed in a distributive, decentralized model.

For each function, the best structure falls somewhere on a continuum between a totally centralized model and a totally decentralized model:

- *Centralized.* Most or all leadership is consolidated at the regional level with limited leadership retained at the site level.
- *Decentralized.* Leadership is required at each site; few opportunities are available to centralize.
- *Partially centralized.* A mix of centralized and decentralized leaders is optimal. For example, certain subregional responsibilities may require leadership to be spread across two or three sites on the basis of proximity or other factors.

Deciding what structure works best for a function requires consideration of multiple criteria. Exhibit 6.2 is an example of factors to consider when redesigning the leadership structure. The collaborative team should rate each function or program against the criteria and determine where on the centralization continuum the programs tend to fall.

The conclusions reached through this exercise enable the team to set expectations and management restructuring targets for each

Exhibit 6.2: Decision Criteria for System Management Restructuring

Criteria	Supports a Decentralized Model	Supports a Partially Centralized Model	Supports a Centralized Model
Regulatory requirements	Regulatory or accreditation requirements mandate that each site have a designated person for this role.	No regulatory or accreditation mandates require this role to be designated for each site.	No regulatory or accreditation mandates require this role to be designated for each site.
Site-based direct reporting staff	Site-based direct reports require significant *daily* oversight and face-to-face supervision.	Site-based staff require periodic (weekly) face-to-face interaction with this position. Role blending may require decentralization at some sites.	Site-based direct reports are highly autonomous and do not require significant oversight and supervision; alternatively, direct reports are concentrated at a central location.
Span of control	The span of control for this position is significant at the site level. Further management rationalization will further increase span.	Span-of-control requirements necessitate partial decentralization of management. Decentralization may occur at sites that do not have enough managers to absorb additional staff.	Span of control is not an issue with regionalization.
Interaction with other functions	The role requires *daily* face-to-face interaction with others outside the function or department, including medical staff members, patients and families, and other site leadership.	The role requires periodic (weekly) interaction with others; daily interaction is not required.	The role does not require frequent face-to-face interaction with others outside the function or department.

(continued)

(continued from previous page)

Exhibit 6.2: Decision Criteria for System Management Restructuring

Criteria	Supports a Decentralized Model	Supports a Partially Centralized Model	Supports a Centralized Model
Work standardization	Work process and outcomes are, by nature, highly variable by site for this function; no significant benefits or opportunities are brought to bear by standardizing practices across the region.	Some opportunities are evident to standardize practices; these are best coordinated among a subset of the sites rather than through a region-wide initiative.	Significant opportunities are evident to standardize practices across the region, requiring the help of central leadership to coordinate.
Regional market coordination	The program or department is highly customized to local market conditions; centralization adversely reduces local market responsiveness.	Some centralization is justified across sites in close proximity that have overlapping markets.	Market responsiveness can be better achieved through centralized planning and coordination.
Improved efficiencies	Minimal work redundancies occur across the sites; centralizing this role has no impact on full-time equivalents (FTEs).	Some work redundancies are seen across the sites; partially centralizing this role results in some FTE and cost savings.	Significant work redundancies are seen across the sites; centralizing this role results in FTE and cost savings.
Improved effectiveness	Centralizing leadership has a disparate impact on the quality of services provided.	Centralized leadership has minimal impact on service quality.	Centralized leadership will improve service quality and ensure process and service consistency across the system.

function. In cases where a regional leadership position is established (e.g., regional director of pharmacy services), the collaborative team should identify an individual (internally or externally) to assume the position and charge him with completing the restructuring for that area.

Implementing Management Restructuring

Management restructuring can be a disruptive process that is highly visible to the rest of the organization. Implementing a new leadership structure takes time and should consider the following concerns:

- The leaders selected to head the organization are symbolic of the desired culture and management style going forward.
- Leaders require time to adapt to new roles and reporting relationships.
- Staff may initially react unfavorably to some leadership changes.
- Some system sites and departments perceive management consolidation as a loss of autonomy and influence.
- Departing leaders should be treated with respect and support.
- Severance costs and other associated expenses initially offset some savings generated by restructuring.

LEVER 9: SYSTEM RATIONALIZATION

Regional management restructuring is often a precursor to system-wide program and service rationalization. Part of the impetus for a stand-alone organization to join a health system is to enable cost and productivity improvements that cannot be achieved separately. New additions to a health system create redundancies in programs, departments, and staff positions. Regional leaders are often tasked with identifying and pursuing opportunities in their areas of responsibility to consolidate operations and reduce expenses across the system.

System rationalization is the process by which health systems identify and pursue opportunities to streamline duplicate processes, services, and programs. Specifically, leaders of these initiatives seek to

- drive down operating costs by lowering fixed operating expenses;
- reposition services and programs in the market to improve the organization's competitive position;
- consolidate demand across small, subscale programs; and
- maintain or improve access and services to patients and internal customers of the system.

Part of the drive to improve services is building consistencies across the system in services affecting patients, physicians, and staff. Consolidating human resources policies and systems, for example, is a critical strategy for building a common culture across disparate system entities.

Administrative and Support Services Rationalization

System rationalization can result in significant productivity (as well as capital and supply savings) gains, particularly in support and administrative services that benefit from increased scale. Laboratory services, for example, are often consolidated into a central lab, while small STAT (immediate need) operations are retained at remaining care sites.

Many systems consolidate patient accounts into a central billing office that serves the entire system. Moving from a decentralized to a centralized business office model can generate high productivity gains and improve consistency in the processing of patient accounts and billings.

Exhibit 6.3 identifies some functional areas in which rationalization opportunities are most prevalent in large healthcare systems. The magnitude of opportunity depends on both the size of a program—usually the collective number of full-time equivalent staff (FTEs)—and the degree to which services can be centralized.

The top half of exhibit 6.3 shows functions that have high staffing complements with significant productivity improvement

Exhibit 6.3: Key Functional Opportunities for System Rationalization

	Partial Centralization	Centralization

High Productivity Savings	Laboratory services
	Dietary services
	Human resources
	Materials management
	Patient care
	    administration
		Accounting
		Business office/patient
		    accounts
		Information systems
		Administration
		Patient scheduling and
		    preregistration

Low Productivity Savings	Training and
	    development
	Biomedical engineering
	Infection control
	Linen services
	Physician relations
	Quality assurance
	Foundation and
	    development
	Medical records
		Marketing and planning
		Legal services
		Managed care
		Public relations
		Credentialing
		Transcription

opportunities. The size of the productivity opportunity depends on the relative size of the function, the amount of redundant services across the system, and the benefits that accrue from increased scale.

The two columns represent the degree of centralization that is feasible for the function. Partial centralization means portions of a function remain at each site while the rest is consolidated to a central site. Total centralization consolidates the entire function to a single site that supports the entire system.

Rationalized cost savings accrue from many sources, again depending on the function. These include the following:

- Consolidating redundant management staffing
- Combining administrative support positions
- Rationalizing specialist staff, including those responsible for
  - performance management,
  - decision support and information technology,
  - quality control and improvement,
  - training and development, and
  - other specialized expertise
- Batching workload at a central site to increase scale and lower cost per unit
- Reducing purchased services associated with
  - medical leadership and other professional services,
  - equipment support, and
  - facilities maintenance
- Reducing duplicate supply inventories
- Reducing duplicate facilities, rent, and capital equipment

System rationalization should be planned and executed with a focus on PI. Exhibit 6.4 is a partial example of how one system developed savings targets for its regionalization strategy. The process should include the following steps:

1. Inventory operating expenses and staffing, and summarize the findings by functional area. Ideally, this inventory is compiled by mapping all expenses in the general ledger to a standard expense category and functional classification across all system entities.
2. Set improvement targets (percentage of savings off the combined expense totals) for each functional area. In the example shown in exhibit 6.4, the system set separate targets for labor and nonlabor expense. Each function

Exhibit 6.4: Regionalization Savings Targets for Support and Administrative Services (partial list)

Administrative Support

Category	Total System Paid FTEs	Annual Labor Cost	Annual Nonlabor Cost	Annual Total Cost
Accounting	76.7	$5,000,221	$3,488,405	$8,488,626
Admitting/patient registration	223.5	$9,281,287	$5,602,408	$14,883,696
Biomedical engineering	3.6	$237,946	$18,953,137	$19,191,084
Business office/patient accounts	302.5	$10,854,777	$24,922,712	$35,777,488
Dietary	249.0	$7,147,335	$6,620,853	$13,768,187
Engineering and maintenance	119.5	$7,866,920	$11,945,427	$19,812,347
Environmental services	396.6	$11,931,610	$3,938,531	$15,870,142
Infection control	11.2	$868,063	$4,991	$873,054
Information systems	51.9	$2,266,149	$95,228,278	$97,494,427
Laboratory supplies		$0	$11,663,709	$11,663,709
Laboratory services	665.5	$22,051,293	$12,888,600	$34,939,893
Marketing/public relations	32.2	$1,922,146	$6,402,349	$8,324,495
Personnel	58.2	$3,412,579	$3,454,924	$6,867,503

(continued)

(continued from previous page)

Exhibit 6.4: Regionalization Savings Targets for Support and Administrative Services (partial list)

Administrative Support

Category	Labor Targets				Nonlabor Targets				Total Savings Targets		Notes
	Low %	High %	Low $	High $	Low %	High %	Low $	High $	Low $	High $	
Accounting	10%	15%	$500,022	$750,033	0%	2%	$0	$69,768	$500,022	$819,801	Centralize to system, but assign controllers to key sites.
Admitting/patient registration	10%	15%	$928,129	$1,392,193			$0	$0	$928,129	$1,392,193	Centralize scheduling, authorization.
Biomedical engineering	0%	5%	$0	$11,897	3%	5%	$568,594	$947,657	$568,594	$959,554	Consolidate and renegotiate maintenance contacts, reduce duplicative equipment.
Business office/patient accounts	10%	15%	$1,085,478	$1,628,217	0%	0%	$0	$0	$1,085,478	$1,628,217	Combine remaining functions in central business office.
Dietary	10%	15%	$714,733	$1,072,100	10%	15%	$662,085	$993,128	$1,376,819	$2,065,228	Partial centralization.
Engineering and maintenance	3%	5%	$236,008	$393,346			$0	$0	$236,008	$393,346	Leadership consolidation.
Environmental services	10%	15%	$1,193,161	$1,789,742	10%	15%	$393,853	$590,780	$1,587,014	$2,380,521	Regional leadership consolidation.
Infection control	5%	10%	$43,403	$86,806			$0	$0	$43,403	$86,806	Partial centralization.
Information systems			$0	$0			$0	$0	$0	$0	Centralize to system services.
Laboratory supplies			$0	$0	5%	10%	$583,185	$1,166,371	$583,185	$1,166,371	Improve reagent and supply utilization through larger batch processing.
Laboratory services	7%	10%	$1,543,591	$2,205,129			$0	$0	$1,543,591	$2,205,129	Central laboratory + small labs at each site.
Marketing/public relations	10%	15%	$192,215	$288,322			$0	$0	$192,215	$288,322	Centralize to system services.
Personnel			$0	$0			$0	$0	$0	$0	Centralize to system services.

(continued)

(continued from previous page)

Exhibit 6.4: Regionalization Savings Targets for Support and Administrative Services (partial list)

Administrative Support

Category	Percent of Opportunity				$ Opportunity				Notes
	Fiscal Year (FY) 2014	FY 2015	FY 2016	FY 2017	FY 2014	FY 2015	FY 2016	FY 2017	
Accounting	30%	50%	70%	90%	$197,974	$329,956	$461,938	$593,921	
Admitting/patient registration	30%	50%	70%	90%	$348,048	$580,080	$812,113	$1,044,145	Central scheduling.
Biomedical engineering	30%	50%	70%	90%	$229,222	$382,037	$534,852	$687,667	Should see some reduction in maintenance resulting from clinical portfolio consolidation.
Business office/patient accounts	30%	50%	70%	90%	$407,054	$678,424	$949,793	$1,221,162	Determine if duplication occurs with other services.
Dietary	30%	50%	70%	90%	$516,307	$860,512	$1,204,716	$1,548,921	Oursource all? Combine food purchasing.
Engineering and maintenance	30%	50%	70%	90%	$94,403	$157,338	$220,274	$283,209	
Environmental services	30%	50%	70%	90%	$595,130	$991,884	$1,388,637	$1,785,391	Outsource all?
Infection control	30%	50%	70%	90%	$19,531	$32,552	$45,573	$58,594	
Information systems	30%	50%	70%	90%	$0	$0	$0	$0	Depends on reduction in home office's allocated costs.
Laboratory supplies	30%	50%	70%	90%	$262,433	$437,389	$612,345	$787,300	
Laboratory services	30%	50%	70%	90%	$562,308	$937,180	$1,312,052	$1,686,924	
Marketing/public relations	30%	50%	70%	90%	$72,080	$120,134	$168,188	$216,241	
Personnel	30%	50%	70%	90%	$0	$0	$0	$0	

Note: FTE = full-time equivalent; FY = fiscal year.

has a range of estimated opportunity, based in part on the amount of duplicated fixed costs. Assumptions and targets can be validated using external benchmarking data.

3. Determine a timeline and sequencing for implementing rationalization in each functional area. Regionalization is a multiyear process. The amount of accrued savings depends on implementation speed and the prioritization of those areas with the highest savings opportunities.

Clinical Services Rationalization

Clinical service rationalization combines the patient volumes of subscale programs into fewer, larger programs. In addition to expense savings, larger-scale programs can build staff proficiency and improve patient safety and clinical outcomes.

For most regional healthcare systems, clinical consolidation focuses on a small number of specialty programs with high, fixed costs such as the following:

- Behavioral health services
- Pediatrics
- Obstetrics
- Inpatient rehabilitation
- Open heart programs
- Neurosurgery programs
- Specialty clinics

Clinical rationalization decisions are more complex than those related to administration and support services because clinical rationalization usually carries particular market risks. Displaced physicians may not support a move to a new location. Likewise, the local patient population may go to a local competitor rather than travel to the new site. Any clinical service rationalization decisions must weigh the benefits with the risk of losing patients and alienating some providers.

LEVER 10: SERVICE REDEPLOYMENT

Cross-functional process design frequently encounters issues related to resource placement. Service deployment is the physical relocation of staff, equipment, and other resources closer to where services are most needed. Moving resources to the point of demand can yield several operational benefits, such as the following:

- Improved service response time for patients and internal customers
- Reduced travel time for staff
- Reduced frequency of patient transports
- Reduced service scheduling and coordination time for caregivers and other staff
- Increased opportunities for developing multiskilled roles
- Enhanced opportunity to rationalize management resources

Service redeployment can occur on a small, intradepartmental basis; among several departments; or across health system entities and markets.

Service Redeployment in a Hospital

Despite the many changes in healthcare over the years, hospital organizational structures have remained fundamentally the same. Hospitals are historically designed to support service centralization. The goal of centralization is to optimize the utilization of staffing and equipment in laboratory, medical imaging, surgery, and other service areas. An artifact of compartmentalization and centralization is the distancing of services and resources from the point of care. This separation results in the need to add infrastructure and increase travel and service coordination, which offsets many of the efficiency gains of centralization.

Redeploying centralized ancillary and support staff can, under certain conditions, improve service and cost performance. Different degrees of service redeployment are feasible in a hospital setting; examples are shown in exhibit 6.5.

Several factors and constraints determine the financial feasibility of service redeployment, including the following:

- *Concentrated consumption.* Demand for the activity occurring at the point of service must be sufficient to make redeployment rational. Infrequently performed tasks have little impact on operations and are generally poor candidates for redeployment.
- *Proficiency requirements.* A redeployed task must be performed with enough frequency to maintain the competencies of the staff who are responsible for service delivery. Managers need to understand the demand for these tasks and how demand varies by hour of day and day of week.
- *Licensure and contract constraints.* Redeployment design must take place within licensure requirements and any labor contract limitations.
- *Capital constraints.* Some service redeployment decisions may require facility redesign or additional equipment. Managers must account for these investments when evaluating the feasibility of redeployment options.

Service redeployment often coincides with role redesign and multiskilled staff. The case example at the end of this chapter demonstrates how one organization created a multiskilled, unit-based service associate position by combining tasks formerly provided by a number of central support services staff.

Exhibit 6.5: Alternative Deployment Strategies

Deployment Strategy	Definition	Examples
Centralized	Services are provided entirely from a single area or department.	• Centralized patient transportation pool • Traditional centralized models for support services • Centralized phlebotomy team
Assigned	Staff report to a central department but are assigned to specific departments, zones, or facilities.	• Deployment of pharmacists to satellite stations that serve one or more departments • Reassignment of a portion of a central transportation pool to medical imaging to cover peak demand times • Location of STAT laboratory services in an emergency department
Integrated	A role formally residing in a centralized department is permanently deployed to a new area and becomes part of that area's work team and operating budget.	• Deployment of a support role to provide support services on nursing units • Redeployment of environmental services staff to operating room staff membership, with expanded support responsibilities
Multiskilled	Specific tasks that were previously provided by a central department are redeployed and added to existing roles in the receiving department.	• Reassignment of phlebotomist functions from a central pool to acute caregivers • Reassignment of some basic respiratory therapy tasks to acute caregivers • Initiation of point-of-care lab testing

System-Level Redeployment

System-level redeployment is the process by which system leaders determine, at the task level, how centralized administrative and support services are best distributed across system entities. Multiple factors influence service redeployment decisions in a healthcare system, including the following:

- The geographic dispersion of system entities
- The need for face-to-face service and interaction with local staff
- The need to customize services for some entities and geographies versus the need to standardize services across the system
- The costs of redundant staffing and duplicate resources at all sites versus rationalzing across multiple entities

Leaders must weigh the pros and cons of centralization on a function-by-function basis. For example, decision and financial support services are functions that, in multientity health systems, are often centralized into a corporate service. A centralized model usually co-locates all managers and analysts in a finance operations center. Typically, they are organized by function relating to the work performed (e.g., budget, decision support systems, financial analysis). This approach has strengths and limitations.

- Pros:
  - Direct oversight of financial leaders is enabled.
  - Resources are pooled in one area with the ability to reassign tasks to members as the workload changes.
  - Cross-training allows for coverage during absences.
  - Standardization in technical systems (e.g., decision support systems, benchmarking sources), accounting practices, and financial reporting is improved.

- Cons:
  - The links among individual operating units can be tenuous and unresponsive to support needs.
  - Groups may become insular and resentful of special requests.
  - Some operating units may seek alternative internal and external resources to meet analytic needs.

A decentralized model may place analysts in a direct reporting relationship with clinical leaders or single-care-site managers. They are tasked with providing information for analysis and decision making for the assigned areas. Staff may be located either at their assigned sites or with other analysts. They manage all financial functions for their areas (e.g., budget, decision support). Typically, this model uses a smaller, more central organization to oversee decision support systems, financial systems, and benchmarking input.

As with centralization, a decentralized model comes with advantages and disadvantages.

- Pros:
  - Support for site needs is responsive. Anticipation of information needs is improved.
  - Analysts are linked directly to operating units, creating a deep knowledge of issues and opportunities.
  - A decentralized model works well with a multiskilled role design.
- Cons:
  - Resources are distributed so aggregation around large projects takes increased effort.
  - Financial accountability and control are lessened.
  - Adherence to analytic standards requires increased monitoring.
  - Career paths are less obvious than in a centralized model.

The optimal degree of centralization is usually a combination of centralized staffing and tasks and decentralized resources physically deployed to multiple operating units.

Exhibit 6.6 is an example of how a regional healthcare system implemented a task-level deployment strategy for human resource services. Each entity operates an on-site office to support local staff recruitment and development and to provide basic personnel services to entity staff. Every office is tailored to the unique needs of each entity and reports to a central system human resources office.

The central office sets human resource policy, administers compensation and payroll services, and performs benefits administration services for the system. The following case example illlustrates a deployment strategy that strikes a balance between local service needs and system requirements while achieving policy uniformity and efficiency across the system.

CASE EXAMPLE: REDEPLOYING SUPPORT SERVICES

A community hospital was experiencing multiple issues related to support services for its acute care operations. Specifically, the organization had

- slow turnaround times for inpatient room turnover,
- low patient satisfaction survey scores for room cleanliness and meal delivery,
- low employee satisfaction among support services personnel,
- excessive time spent by caregivers on support-related activities, and
- a need to improve labor productivity and cost performance.

Exhibit 6.6: Regional Deployment Strategy for Human Resources

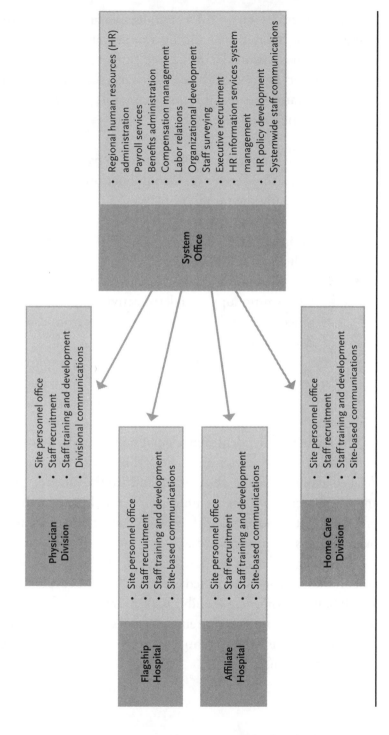

System Office
- Regional human resources (HR) administration
- Payroll services
- Benefits administration
- Compensation management
- Labor relations
- Organizational development
- Staff surveying
- Executive recruitment
- HR information services system management
- HR policy development
- Systemwide staff communications

Physician Division
- Site personnel office
- Staff recruitment
- Staff training and development
- Divisional communications

Flagship Hospital
- Site personnel office
- Staff recruitment
- Staff training and development
- Site-based communications

Affiliate Hospital
- Site personnel office
- Staff recruitment
- Staff training and development
- Site-based communications

Home Care Division
- Site personnel office
- Staff recruitment
- Staff training and development
- Site-based communications

System executives chartered a multidisciplinary collaborative team to evaluate the feasibility of adding a multiskilled service associate role. The team envisioned a unit-based support role that combined unit housekeeping tasks with select dietary, maintenance, supply, and transportation responsibilities. The improvement goals of the project were the following:

- Improve support services provided to patients by
    - increasing service turnaround performance,
    - reducing the number of "faces" a patient encounters during his or her stay,
    - improving the effectiveness of work performed, and
    - reducing staff idle time.
- Reduce the amount of time caregivers spend on
    - performing support-related activities and
    - scheduling and coordinating services from central departments.
- Improve the satisfaction of support service employees and caregivers.
- Improve patient satisfaction with support services.

The team initially identified a list of support tasks that were candidate roles for the service associate (exhibit 6.7). By conducting a detailed activity analysis, the team quantified the time requirements and frequencies by nursing unit. The team also rated the degree of deferrability associated with each task and the requirements for maintaining staff proficiencies.

Next, the team rated the potential deployment of each functional area on the basis of the expected efficiencies from redeployment and a multiskilled workforce (exhibit 6.8). From this information, the team identified staffing requirements and estimated the anticipated productivity gains. The potential sources of improvement derived from the following:

Exhibit 6.7: Support Service Activities by Area

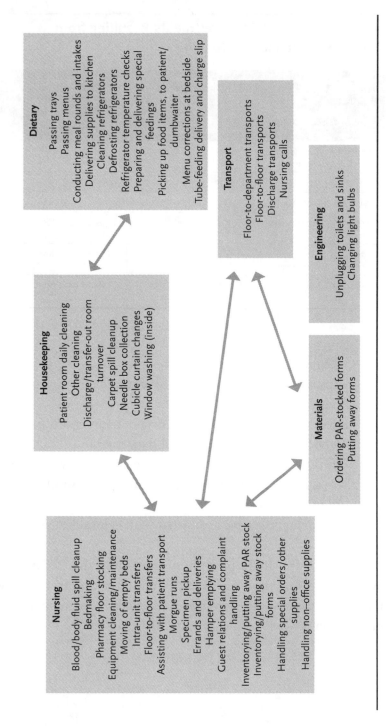

Dietary

Passing trays
Passing menus
Conducting meal rounds and intakes
Delivering supplies to kitchen
Cleaning refrigerators
Defrosting refrigerators
Refrigerator temperature checks
Preparing and delivering special feedings
Picking up food items, to patient/dumbwaiter
Menu corrections at bedside
Tube-feeding delivery and charge slip

Housekeeping

Patient room daily cleaning
Other cleaning
Discharge/transfer-out room turnover
Carpet spill cleanup
Needle box collection
Cubicle curtain changes
Window washing (inside)

Transport

Floor-to-department transports
Floor-to-floor transports
Discharge transports
Nursing calls

Engineering

Unplugging toilets and sinks
Changing light bulbs

Materials

Ordering PAR-stocked forms
Putting away forms

Nursing

Blood/body fluid spill cleanup
Bedmaking
Pharmacy floor stocking
Equipment cleaning/maintenance
Moving of empty beds
Intra-unit transfers
Floor-to-floor transfers
Assisting with patient transport
Morgue runs
Specimen pickup
Errands and deliveries
Hamper emptying
Guest relations and complaint handling
Inventorying/putting away PAR stock
Inventorying/putting away stock forms
Handling special orders/other supplies
Handling non-office supplies

Exhibit 6.8: Potential Improvements Resulting from Redeployment and Multiskilling

Functional Area	Redeployment			Multiskilling		
	Reduced Travel Time?	Rationalized Management?	Reduced Nurse Coordination/ Scheduling?	Parallel Processing?	Eliminated Tasks?	Reduced Downtime?
Housekeeping	Some (discharge team)	Some	Yes	Yes	Some	No
Transport	Yes	Yes	Yes	Yes	Yes	Yes
Engineering	Yes	No	Yes	Yes	No	No
Materials management	Some (between units)	No	Yes	Yes	Yes	No
Dietary	Some (between units)	No	Yes	Some	No	No
Nursing	N/A	N/A	N/A	Yes	Yes	No

- Reducing travel time for staff
- Lowering managerial resource requirements (in some central departments)
- Reducing the time nurse managers spent coordinating services provided by a central department
- Improving the ability to combine new tasks with other tasks at the point of service (parallel processing)
- Eliminating nonvalue tasks
- Reducing idle time associated with centralized services

Results from the implementation showed that redeployment and multiskilling produced a 12 percent reduction in FTEs. More important, the new position improved service turnaround times and satisfaction levels for patients and unit-based staff.

CHAPTER 7

Optimizing Nonlabor Expenses

MEDICAL SUPPLIES TYPICALLY account for 15 to 20 percent of the average hospital's operating expenses and are a component of most departmental budgets. For this reason, performance improvement (PI) initiatives frequently include a focus on spending for supplies, purchased services, and other nonlabor expense categories.

The primary supply categories for a health system include the following:

- Consumable medical supplies for nursing, physician offices, and other routine patient care areas
- Implants, endomechanical devices, and other supplies in surgery
- Implants and supplies for invasive cardiac services
- Reagents and other clinical laboratory supplies
- Imaging supplies
- Pharmaceuticals
- Food and nutritional products
- Blood and blood products
- Laundry and linen supplies
- Office supplies and forms

Exhibit 7.1 is example of the annual supply expenditures for a large, multihospital system and the relative proportion of spending by category.

As demonstrated in this example, pharmaceuticals, surgery supplies, and routine medical supplies account for nearly three quarters of a typical hospital system's supply budget. As such, most cost improvement opportunities reside in these three supply categories.

SUPPLY STRATEGIES

Clinicians can spend considerable time on supply-related activities, including inventory management, searching for supplies and equipment, cleaning and sterilizing equipment, and charging for supply usage. Excessive inventories increase holding costs and require additional staffing for supply receiving, storage, and distribution.

Exhibit 7.1: Example of Annual Supply Expenses for a Multihospital System

Supply Category	Annual Spend	Total Supply Spend
Pharmaceuticals	$52,537,902	28%
Consumable medical supplies	$45,323,720	24%
Surgical supplies	$39,609,070	21%
Cardiac supplies (catheterization lab)	$12,551,743	7%
Food and nutrition	$10,364,809	6%
Laboratory supplies	$9,508,327	5%
Blood products	$7,754,948	4%
Medical imaging supplies	$4,861,975	3%
Office supplies and forms	$4,406,083	2%
Annual total	**$186,918,577**	

From a labor productivity perspective, healthcare managers should focus on supply strategies that

- simplify and improve supply chain processes to minimize the time spent by clinical staff to purchase items;
- locate high-usage supply items at the point of care to minimize the time spent by clinical staff to search for needed items;
- leverage technologies (e.g., automated supply cabinets, bar coding) to simplify supply inventory management, asset tracking, and patient charging;
- minimize on-hand inventories that drive up holding costs and materials management staffing; and
- maintain patient care equipment to minimize its rate of malfunction and delays in patient care resulting from the absence of equipment that has not yet been replaced.

Purchasing Medical Products

Medical products generally fall within one of two broad classes:

- *Commodities*—including many consumable medical and surgical routine items, office supplies, and most food and nutrition products
- *Noncommodities*—including items that have no therapeutic equivalent; supplies that are required to operate specific equipment; and branded items, such as surgical implants, that are used according to physicians' individual preferences

Hospitals purchase most commodity and some noncommodity supplies through national group purchasing organizations (GPOs) and distributers. Hospitals control supply expenditures, in part, through product standardization and the maximization of compliance with GPO agreements. Organizations with purchasing leverage (e.g., large scale, with market share dominance) contract directly with manufacturers for implants and other non-commodity products. Additionally, some systems participate in regional purchasing cooperatives focused on obtaining favorable pricing for high-volume commodity supplies. The success of these regional programs to negotiate favorable pricing depends on how effectively the cooperative drives standardization and compliance across member organizations.

Distributors are responsible for reselling and delivering pharmaceuticals, medical supplies, and device-related products to hospitals, physician offices, and other providers. Distributors serve an intermediary role between customer needs and the manufacturers, particularly in managing and physically delivering supplies.

Distributors may influence caregiver product selection in cases where the distributor has a strategic marketing arrangement with a manufacturer. Some distributors carry private-label products of their own, which compete with those of other manufacturers. Distributors use some of the same marketing practices that manufacturers do, though the extent of use and level of investment are considerably smaller.

STRATEGIES RELATED TO MEDICAL DEVICES

Medical devices are a critical component of the diagnostic and interventional procedures performed by physicians and other caregivers. Device manufacturers produce a wide array of consumable supplies, procedural devices, and diagnostic equipment. Products include orthopedic implants, diagnostic imaging equipment, medical and surgical instruments, interventional cardiology products, and patient monitoring devices. These products often have short life cycles, requiring a continuing feedback loop with providers to fuel ongoing innovation and continuous improvement.

Health systems employ similar efforts to standardize high-cost medical devices used in surgery, invasive cardiac care, and diagnostic services. Product selection can, in many cases, determine when a procedure is profitable or unprofitable for organizations. For example, orthopedic implants can account for 50 percent or more of the total cost for total joint replacement surgery, depending on the brand and category of implant used.

Physicians must understand new technology and the specific techniques for using it. For this reason, physicians are heavily recruited by device manufacturers to serve as trainers and instructors to other physicians when a new product is introduced to the market. Medical device sales representatives enjoy high visibility with physicians and hospital staff, and they frequently assist in using their company's products in surgery and other clinical settings.

TACTICS FOR MANAGING PHARMACEUTICAL EXPENSES

Pharmaceuticals represent one of the highest growth expense categories for health systems. Inpatient drug spending growth increases more than 10 percent per year, driven primarily by unit pricing increases (NORC at the University of Chicago 2016). Costs are driven by the continuous introduction of new branded drugs. Much of this increase occurs in specialty drug categories, including

- antivirals,
- antineoplastics,
- hematinics and blood stimulators, and
- antiarthritics.

Most healthcare systems purchase pharmaceuticals through national contracts with GPOs. Pharmacy cost improvement opportunities in a health system are found in utilization control, standardization, and formulary management. Physicians have primary responsibility for selecting the drugs and medical devices used in patient care. Consequently, health systems must work closely with the medical staff to rein in drug utilization and prescribing variation.

Addressing Physician Preferences

Hospitals continuously evaluate and manage the number of medical supply line items and pharmaceuticals used in their organization. The most challenging items are physician preference items (PPIs), to which a doctor builds loyalty over time. This preference for particular brands or items occurs primarily with regard to medical devices and is influenced by manufacturers' relationships with surgeons, cardiologists, and other specialists.

Physician product awareness is shaped by three primary factors:

- *Provider education.* Physicians learn about new products and research from medical journals, educational conferences (continuing medical education and company-sponsored training), and other practitioners. Indirect advertising can also be considered educational.
- *Patient preference.* Increasingly, manufacturers use direct-to-consumer advertising to build consumer awareness of new drugs and devices. Patients may thereby influence physicians in prescribing and device selection.
- *Relationships.* This preference category represents any direct financial relationships between providers and companies, including equity interest, consulting relationships, and sponsorship of clinical trials.

Vendors frequently provide pricing incentives to encourage health systems to consolidate purchasing in product categories. In many cases, taking advantage of these promotions requires health systems to convince physicians to change vendors. The pressure to lower PPI pricing increases as reimbursement shifts to case-based and bundled pricing. Health system supply chain leaders must work closely with affiliated physicians to manage the costs and utilization of PPI supplies.

LEVER 11: NONLABOR OPTIMIZATION

Nonlabor optimization seeks to lower costs associated with the procurement, receiving, storage, and distribution of supplies and equipment and to manage purchased service expenditures. Before launching a nonlabor initiative, leaders should assess the organization's supply chain processes and systems regarding the following:

- Procurement processes and protocols
- Distribution and inventory management performance
- Supply expense budgeting and control processes
- Contract monitoring and compliance
- Purchasing rebate management
- Processes for local supplier negotiation
- Processes for engaging physicians in product evaluation
- Product standardization and value analysis

The scope of a nonlabor PI initiative varies from one to the next, but it often includes all supply categories, pharmaceuticals, and purchased services. The composition of the collaborative PI team should reflect the functional areas under the team scope. For large, multisite supply chain initiatives, subteams can be assigned to specific supply categories (e.g., pharmacy team, surgical supply team, laboratory supply team).

SUPPLY CHAIN IMPROVEMENT

The diversity and nature of supply categories requires different improvement strategies than those used for other operational improvements. As shown in exhibit 7.2, cost improvements in the supply chain focus on lowering the cost per unit purchased, reducing the demand and consumption of supplies, and controlling inventory and associated holding costs. In addition, pharmaceutical and purchased service expenses must be managed.

Lowering Unit Pricing

Nonlabor PI teams should first seek to identify opportunities to lower the unit costs associated with high-volume and high-spend products and categories. This reduction can be achieved through several means, such as the following:

- *Price renegotiation.* GPOs and purchasing cooperatives perform pricing negotiations for most hospital products. Member organizations have a significant economic incentive to maximize compliance with their GPO contracts. A supply chain team should identify "off-contract" purchasing and determine if the item is covered under a group contract. For some product categories, such as surgical implants, food, and office supplies, health systems may obtain better pricing through local negotiation.
- *Market consolidation.* Supply manufacturers frequently offer tiered pricing for consumable medical products. Pricing is usually based on the percentage of total spend in a product category for a single supplier, with a higher percentage corresponding to lower unit pricing. Supply teams should review compliance reports and determine if additional savings can accrue by shifting additional market share to a lower-cost supplier.
- *Pricing constructs.* Pricing constructs are used to establish fixed prices for product categories supplied by multiple vendors. Constructs are useful for reducing costs associated with high-cost PPI supply categories, such as implants

Exhibit 7.2: Supply Chain Improvement Strategies

	Improvement Strategy	Definition	Example	Primarily Applicable to	
				Commodity Items	Noncommodity Items
Lower Unit Pricing	Price renegotiation	Reduce unit pricing through renegotiation or adoption of new GPO contracts (no change in volume or market shift).	Adopt the GPO's new contract for contrast media.	X	X
	Market consolidation	Reduce the number of vendors for a product category to take advantage of better tiered pricing.	Reduce the number of stent vendors from 4 to 2.		X
	Pricing construct	Negotiate a fixed ceiling price for a product category that all vendors must meet.	Pricing constructs for orthopedic implants.		X
	Product change-out	Switch out a product with a comparable, lower-cost substitute.	Change suppliers for commodity products.	X	
Reduce Demand	Reduced utilization	Reduce consumption of products based on changes in practice protocols or other utilization improvements.	Change IV set change-outs from 72 to 96 hours.	X	
	Demand matching	Implement protocols to control the use of high-cost products when lower-cost products are therapeutically equivalent.	Therapeutic guidelines for antibiotic usage.		X
	Waste reduction	Reduce the incidence of products that are discarded without use.	Reconfigure suture kits to eliminate items that are rarely used.	X	X
	Reprocessing	Use remanufactured products.	Use reconditioned pulse oximeters in patient care areas.		X
Reduce Holding Costs	Inventory management	Reduce the amount of on-hand inventory.	Consignment inventory, lower loss and waste.	X	X

Note: GPO = group purchasing organization; IV = intravenous.

for orthopedic and spine procedures. Construct pricing enables the organization to exercise price control while allowing physicians to use their vendor of preference.

- *Product change-outs.* Teams may identify opportunities to replace items with an equivalent product from a different vendor. This strategy is common with commodity products and can often take place with minimal disruption and communication.

Reducing Demand

In addition to lowering the unit cost for supplies, organizations can reduce the number of supply units consumed. This reduction can be achieved in the following ways:

- *Reduced utilization.* Lowering the supply expense per case or per ambulatory visit. Some examples include
  - reducing inpatient length of stay to decrease the use of routine consumable medical supplies;
  - standardizing order sets to drive a significant number of orders for testing, supplies, and pharmaceuticals by reviewing order sets to identify cases that produce unnecessary overutilization;
  - introducing clinical practice protocols to regulate the use of many medical supplies by reviewing existing protocols for high-volume patient care tasks to determine if practices result in excessive supply utilization (e.g., changing the frequency of intravenous [IV] set change-outs from 72 hours to 96 hours, thereby substantially reducing supply expenses without reducing quality of care); and
  - developing protocols for the effective utilization of blood and IV immunoglobulin products.

- *Demand matching.* Using less costly implants in cases where the medical need does not warrant an expensive product. Examples include
  - cardiac stents (bare metal versus drug eluting),
  - cardiac rhythm management devices, and
  - orthopedic implants (low demand versus high demand).
- *Waste reduction.* Reducing the amount of product that is discarded without being used. Such waste occurs frequently in surgical services and is driven by vendor packaging of procedure kits, surgeon's judgment, inaccurate PPIs, and other factors.
- *Reprocessing.* Using an outside service to reprocess certain medical devices for reuse. Reprocessed devices have efficacy levels that are equivalent to new products at considerably lower unit costs. Examples include
  - endoscopic trocars,
  - pulse oximeters,
  - compression devices,
  - electrophysiology catheters,
  - laparoscopes, and
  - tourniquet cuffs.

Controlling Inventory Holding Costs

Inventory holding costs may present an additional opportunity for some organizations to initiate PI. Supply inventories for most hospitals have diminished in recent years because of daily shipments from supply distributors and the use of consignment inventory, and because other strategies that minimize on-hand supplies are more common than in the past. From a cost reduction perspective, lowering on-hand inventory levels can reduce waste associated with expired or lost supplies.

Managing Pharmaceutical Expenses

Drug and pharmacy-related expenses are a common component of supply chain improvement initiatives and clinical utilization projects. Often, subteams are assigned to focus on the unique supply and demand issues associated with pharmaceuticals. These initiatives are usually headed by a pharmacy leader with support from clinical pharmacists, materials management staff, and physicians.

As shown in exhibit 7.3, various levels of interventions are available to reduce pharmaceutical costs, including the following:

- *Cost per drug.* These strategies are designed to reduce the unit prices of drugs. They include complying with GPO contracts, replacing brand drugs with generic equivalents when feasible, selecting lower-cost brand drugs when therapeutically equivalent options are available, and other interventions.

Exhibit 7.3 Pharmaceutical Cost Interventions

Level of Cost Improvement	Examples
Cost per drug	• Group purchasing • Consolidate vendors • Generic substitution • Drug use and evaluation • Drug prep and compounding • Drug route (e.g., IV to oral)
Cost per therapeutic class	• Therapeutic class review • Therapeutic interchange and substitution • Antibiotic stewardship
Cost per case	• Standard order sets and care plans • Clinical pharmacist consultation and review
Cost per covered population	• Lower prescription rates and total drug expenses per member per month

- *Cost per therapeutic class.* This approach helps teams manage total spending in a class of drugs by identifying alternative, less costly drugs and by managing physician ordering through formulary controls and automatic substitution. In recent years, for example, many health systems have instituted stewardship programs to manage costs and utilization associated with antibiotics.
- *Cost per case.* These initiatives aim to reduce drug expenses for inpatient cases. This reduction is achieved through the effective design of standard order sets for pharmaceuticals and physician consultative services provided by clinical pharmacists.
- *Cost per covered population.* As population health management grows in prevalence, more health systems will need to focus on managing the utilization and costs of drugs for patients across the care continuum.

Reducing Purchased Service Expenses

Nonlabor collaborative teams often evaluate purchased service expenses to identify cost improvement opportunities. Purchased services can represent 10 to 15 percent of a system's operating budget. Some common examples of purchased services include the following:

- Biomedical maintenance and repair services
- Contracted labor
- Support services contracting for
  - environmental services,
  - dietary services, and
  - laundry and linen services
- Legal and other consulting fees
- Outside laboratory referral services and blood processing fees

- Revenue collection services
- Physician services
- Building construction and renovation services

The amount a system spends on purchased services depends, in large part, on the financial viability of and organizational support for service outsourcing. For example, biomedical maintenance services can be provided by an internal biomedical team, by an external original equipment manufacturer agreement, or through some combination of these approaches. The best solution for an organization depends on multiple factors, including the size of the organization, its equipment inventory, and its ability to attract and retain qualified staff for employment in these roles.

Healthcare systems typically contract with physician groups and individuals to provide professional services, including emergency care, imaging services, and anesthesia coverage. Organizations also contract with individuals to serve in clinical program leadership and other positions. The number of contracts to track and manage can be considerable. Health system executives should continuously monitor contract compliance and terms to identify overspending or cases where services are no longer required or can be scaled back.

Specifically, purchased service expenses can be reduced through numerous interventions, including the following:

- Renegotiating existing service contracts to improve terms and pricing
- Eliminating outsourced services that can be provided more effectively in-house
- Auditing and improving contract compliance from current service providers
- Reducing expenditures on discretionary spending for consulting, legal services, marketing and public relations, and other professional services

CHAPTER 8

Improving Quality and Clinical Utilization

THE INCREASING ADOPTION of value-based reimbursement strategies underscores the high variation and prevalence of unnecessary care and resource consumption that exists in the US healthcare system. Value-based healthcare compels providers to optimize clinical outcomes while minimizing unnecessary clinical service utilization and costs. Overutilization drives up medical costs and increases risks for patients (Emanuel and Fuchs 2008).

Significant cost and quality variation occurs among providers in health systems and across organizations and regions. Exhibit 8.1 is a comparison of Medicare inpatient costs and quality performance for large Oklahoma hospitals. As this example demonstrates, cost of care has little positive correlation with quality outcomes. For many markets, high-quality organizations often are the lowest-cost performers. In many cases, quality improvement can reduce operating expenses, lower costs for patients and payers, and increase provider operating margins.

For most health systems, clinical quality and utilization represent the greatest sources of waste reduction and long-term performance improvement (PI). Most provider organizations have significant opportunities to lower healthcare costs and improve outcomes by reducing the incidence of the following occurrences:

- Clinically unnecessary or redundant testing, therapies, and procedures
- Unnecessary admissions and readmissions
- The overprescribing of drugs and other pharmaceuticals
- Unnecessary emergency department visits
- Excessive inpatient length of stay (LOS)
- Off-quality events

Clinical utilization and quality improvements can be difficult to achieve and sustain. Healthcare organizations and clinicians seeking

---

Exhibit 8.1: Cost and Quality Comparisons—Oklahoma Medicare Cases

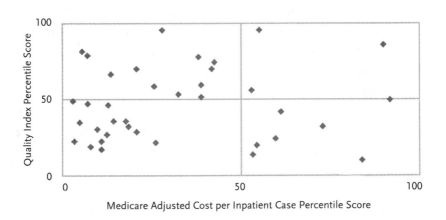

Source: Data from Medicare Provider and Analysis Review (MedPAR) files.

Note: Each diamond represents a separate acute care facility. Organizations in this analysis have 600 or more inpatient Medicare cases per year. Cost per case (*x*-axis) was computed on the basis of analysis of MedPAR files for inpatient discharges and Medicare cost reporting data for 2013 and by applying a cost-to-charges ratio costing methodology. Cost per discharge amounts were adjusted by case mix index and the Medicare wage index. The quality index percentile score (*y*-axis) is a composite score of an organization's performance on 24 process-of-care indicators for the same period.

clinical improvement typically encounter myriad challenges, such as the following:

- Clinical utilization and quality improvements typically take time to research and identify to determine specific interventions. Thus, identifying appropriate, evidence-based practices can be challenging for many clinical processes.
- Opportunities are often spread across most service lines, patient populations, and providers.
- A high degree of cost and outcomes variation is often seen among practitioners providing the same service or procedure.
- Most health systems encounter some degree of resistance from physicians and caregivers when standardizing care across providers and sites.

Healthcare organizations must solicit the support and active involvement of physicians in leading clinical improvement initiatives. Physicians and other clinicians care about quality and outcomes and reducing harm to patients. Cost improvements, while desirable, cannot be the primary driver of change. Clinical performance improvement must be pursued as a means for improving patient care and preserving patient safety.

As changes are identified, organizations need clinician support to ensure successful implementation and widespread adoption. As a starting point, formal leaders and groups (e.g., the chief medical officer [CMO], the medical executive committee, program chairs) must provide effective leadership in setting priorities and goals, evaluating clinical performance, and leading PI initiatives. These leaders in turn must be supported with effective

- data and performance measurement systems,
- processes for identifying and prioritizing clinical improvement initiatives,

- improvement frameworks and approaches that engage all key stakeholders (e.g., medical staff, nursing, pharmacy department),
- governance processes and structure that help guide decision making, and
- incentive systems that reinforce quality and utilization improvement across the organization.

Starting with Data

Clinical quality and utilization improvement initiatives require an informational foundation that is reliable and trusted by leaders and clinical staff. High-performing organizations invest in data and decision support systems that provide the information necessary to assist leaders and collaborative teams.

To construct a strong informational foundation, health systems require proficiencies in several areas:

- An effective cost accounting system for accurately measuring direct costs and profitability by diagnosis-related group (DRG) for inpatient services. The system should provide an accurate breakdown of costs by intermediate service component (e.g., nursing, pharmacy, operating room). Ideally, organizations should institute micro-cost accounting systems that accurately measure the direct expenses associated with each case. Absent a detailed costing system, organizations can employ a cost-to-charges ratio methodology, which provides a reasonable estimate of costs.
- Systems for measuring utilization, direct costs, and profitability for key outpatient and ambulatory services.
- Tracking and reporting of inpatient LOS performance by DRG, physician, and service line.

- Throughput measures for the intensive care unit (ICU) and emergency services, surgery, and acute care areas.
- Systems to measure the performance dimensions of clinical and service quality and patient safety.
- Internal benchmarks to measure clinician variation and external benchmarks to identify and size improvement opportunities.

LEVER 12: OFF-QUALITY IMPROVEMENT

Off-quality improvement pertains to focused interventions designed to improve clinical and service performance outcomes. The goals of these initiatives are to achieve the following:

- Maximized clinical outcomes
- Minimized patient safety incidences and other off-quality events
- Reduced incremental costs incurred with off-quality events
- Improved value-based reimbursement
- Reduced costs associated with litigation and malpractice

Adverse quality and safety events compromise outcomes and patient safety, and they add considerable costs to patient care services. The seminal Institute of Medicine (2001) report *Crossing the Quality Chasm* revealed the urgent need to improve quality of care and patient safety in healthcare delivery.

The incidence of postoperative deep vein thrombosis (DVT), for example, is an issue for many health systems. As shown in exhibit 8.2, one multihospital system had 114 incidences of postoperative DVT out of a total caseload of 19,784 annual surgeries.

The organization found that cases involving patients who experienced DVT had a direct cost per case of nearly $10,000 higher than those without. DVT cases had higher LOS and an average negative

Exhibit 8.2: On-Quality Versus Off-Quality Costs—Surgery Cases with and Without Incidence of Deep Vein Thrombosis (DVT)

	Cases Without DVT	Cases with DVT
Total annual surgery cases	19,670	114
Average direct cost per case	$25,728	$34,077
Operating margin per case	$7,954	–$395
Average length of stay (days)	4.5	6.8
Total excess costs = 114 cases × ($34,077 – $25,728) = $951,786.		
Total excess days = (6.8 – 4.5) × 114 = 262 days.		

contribution margin. The total excess cost of DVT was estimated at nearly $1 million.

Using this methodology, the organization calculated the estimated added costs of other off-quality events (exhibit 8.3). On the basis of this analysis, the organization determined that off-quality events for inpatient services generated an estimated $4 million in additional direct costs. The organization used this information to charter several multidisciplinary collaborative teams focused on lowering the incidence of measures with the highest excess costs.

Quality Performance and Value-Based Reimbursement

Although clinical quality improvement has always been imperative, the industry's move to value-based reimbursement is raising the stakes for providers. PI plans should include provisions for improving patient outcomes and safety to, in part, minimize the financial risks associated with value-based purchasing.

Exhibit 8.3: Calculation of Annual Off-Quality Costs and Excess Patient Days by Patient Safety Indicator

Quality Indicator	Total On-Quality Cases	Total Off-Quality Cases	Off-Quality Excess	Excess Days
Postoperative PE/DVT	19,670	114	$951,786	262
Postoperative respiratory failure	10,148	108	$718,601	270
Accidental puncture/laceration	70,569	135	$534,193	319
Pressure ulcer	18,817	21	$485,053	48
Postoperative sepsis	2,136	33	$447,716	86
Postoperative hemorrhage/ hematoma	19,815	37	$300,369	110
Bloodstream infection—neonates	217	5	$259,888	12
Central venous catheter–related bloodstream infection	53,054	23	$166,877	62
Postoperative physiologic/metabolic derangements	11,659	4	$126,145	3
Iatrogenic pneumothorax	68,317	17	$112,281	45
Postoperative wound dehiscence	2,951	4	$60,595	0
OB trauma—vaginal delivery without instrument	3,678	82	$40,973	157
OB trauma—vaginal delivery with instrument	208	35	$40,202	88
Bilateral cardiac catheterization	2,704	34	$17,614	65
Foreign body left during procedure	2,825	5	$14,312	0
Incidental appendectomy—elderly	1,043	12	$14,003	15
Birth trauma—injury to neonate	6,071	3	$1,250	10
Iatrogenic pneumothorax—neonate	415	0	$0	
Postoperative hip fracture	11,180	0	$0	
Transfusion reaction	125	0	$0	
Total			**$4,291,859**	**1,552**

Note: DVT = deep-vein thrombosis; OB = obstetric; PE = pulmonary embolism.

As the largest payer for hospital-based services, the Centers for Medicare & Medicaid Services (CMS) has taken the industry lead on value-based reimbursement. Two Medicare programs—the Inpatient Value-Based Purchasing (VBP) program and the Hospital Readmissions Reduction Program (HRRP)—are notable.

Medicare Inpatient Value-Based Purchasing Program

The Inpatient VBP program was enacted to reward Medicare providers who demonstrate high quality and achieve high patient satisfaction. For each hospital participating in the Medicare program, a portion of annual payments is held at risk and redistributed based on a set of performance criteria that include the following:

- Mortality and complications
- Healthcare-associated infections
- Patient safety
- Patient experience and satisfaction
- Process-of-care measures
- Efficiency and cost reduction

On the basis of an organization's performance, the total payment from Medicare is greater or less than past reimbursement levels. Low performance in any of these dimensions represents potential focus areas for collaborative teams. Organizations with low patient engagement scores, for example, should launch initiatives to evaluate and improve areas that are consistently rated low by patients on satisfaction surveys. Medicare requires hospitals to administer HCAHPS (the Hospital Consumer Assessment of Healthcare Providers and Systems) survey to measure satisfaction for Medicare beneficiaries (CMS 2014). PI efforts can target one or more of the following areas addressed by the survey:

- Nursing care
- Doctors' care
- Environmental factors
- Discharge instructions

Medicare Hospital Readmissions Reduction Program

The HRRP was instituted by CMS (2017c) to penalize hospitals that have high incidences of patients being readmitted soon after discharge. Under this plan, all Medicare admissions that occur within 30 days of a previous discharge are considered readmissions (excluding planned hospitalizations). Currently, the program focuses on readmissions associated with heart attack, heart failure, pneumonia, chronic obstructive pulmonary disease, elective hip or knee replacement procedures, and coronary artery bypass graft (CABG) surgery.

Organizations with high readmission rates can lower Medicare reimbursement penalties by focusing on multiple processes and issues that lead to unwarranted readmissions. Options may include improving patient discharge planning and instructions, coordinating with post-acute care providers and patients' primary care physicians, and reducing medical complications during patients' initial hospital stay (Kripalani et al. 2014).

Collaborative Teams and Off-Quality Improvement

Clinical quality and safety improvement are often addressed with separate teams or separate initiatives. Patient safety issues, for example, can cross all patient populations and reflect underlying system and process issues that should be addressed through a focused initiative. Health systems frequently employ collaborative teams to correct these off-quality issues. A team's charter may include an economic savings target commensurate with the expected incidence reduction.

Off-quality issues may be a primary focus of a collaborative team or tackled as a component of an initiative aimed at improvement for specific diagnoses or patient populations. Exhibit 8.4 is a graphic representation of a team concerned with improving care and costs associated with pneumonia patients. In addition to looking at cost and utilization issues, the team is tasked with improving the rate of pressure ulcers occurring with pneumonia patients. Also, the team

Exhibit 8.4: Clinical Collaborative Team Scope—Pneumonia Team Example

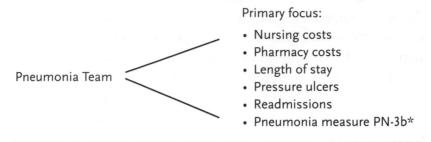

Pneumonia Team

Primary focus:
- Nursing costs
- Pharmacy costs
- Length of stay
- Pressure ulcers
- Readmissions
- Pneumonia measure PN-3b*

*From the Joint Commission Core Measures.

seeks to improve performance in one of the Medicare Core Measures: PN-3B, Blood Cultures Performed in the Emergency Department Prior to Initial Antibiotic Received in Hospital.

Off-quality teams are typically led by a physician or another clinical leader. These groups focus on clinical issues that occur as part of nursing care or processes performed in surgery, labor and delivery, and other procedural areas. The teams' work should be supported by case reviews and other clinical data to identify causal factors and support changes that prevent future occurrences. Organizations need effective surveillance systems in place to monitor quality and safety performance by case and by physician. As off-quality events occur, the organization must employ effective protocols for engaging physicians and improving performance.

LEVER 13: CLINICAL UTILIZATION IMPROVEMENT

The advent of case-based reimbursement, population health mandates, and risk-based contracting compels hospitals to improve acute care cost performance. Any overutilization of care reduces the per case contribution margin for patient care. The term *clinical utilization management* encompasses the myriad improvement strategies healthcare organizations employ to reduce unnecessary or low-value patient care. Lowering acute care service costs represents a significant opportunity for improving financial performance in most health systems.

Armed with benchmark data and premeasured improvement opportunities, organizations can assign multidisciplinary collaborative teams to identify utilization improvement opportunities that lower direct costs per case. Typically, an organization forms a core clinical utilization collaborative team to oversee all clinical improvement initiatives. This team is usually chaired by the CMO or another senior-level executive responsible for clinical operations.

Subteams can be assigned to clinical service lines or key diagnostic categories. A cardiac team, for example, may be assigned responsibility for improvements in procedures and treatments related to acute myocardial infarction, CABG, pacemakers, and cardiac stents. Clinical teams should include relevant and influential physicians and representatives from nursing, pharmacy, imaging, laboratory, rehabilitative services, surgery, and case management.

Before launching clinical utilization teams, the organization should measure and summarize direct costs per case for each DRG and service line and compare performance to industry benchmarks. Exhibit 8.5 is a summary report of the five DRGs associated with CABGs. The analysis provides a cost-per-case breakdown of key components of care, including nursing, cardiac services, surgery, pharmacy, and laboratory. Cost components that exceed peer benchmarks are highlighted. Additional information is provided on LOS performance, and an indicator flags DRGs with significant variation in cost per case among providers.

This kind of analysis is a critical component of the information used to facilitate the work of clinical improvement teams and identify specific opportunities. Clinical utilization improvement can occur at the following levels:

- Component
- Diagnosis

Exhibit 8.5: Component-Level Evaluation for Coronary Artery Bypass Grafting Cases

DRG	DRG Description	No. of Cases for Period	Nursing Services			Ancillary Services								Total	LOS Opportunity	Internal Variation
			General Med–Surg	Intermediate Care	Critical Care	Cardiac Services	Imaging Services	Laboratory Services	Surgical Services	Pharmacy Services	Respiratory Services	Rehab Services	Other			
232	CORONARY BYPASS W PTCA W/O MCC	7	$0	$3,554	$4,355	$3,685	$217	$1,732	$12,388	$2,359	$445	$325	$170	$29,230	4.7	
233	CORONARY BYPASS W CARDIAC CATH W MCC	10	$320	$4,314	$16,143	$1,900	$777	$6,740	$12,432	$11,234	$1,231	$1,539	$3,330	$59,960	111.7	HIGH
234	CORONARY BYPASS W CARDIAC CATH W/O MCC	28	$153	$2,072	$4,279	$1,736	$345	$2,311	$10,756	$2,076	$451	$399	$340	$24,918	43.5	
235	CORONARY BYPASS W/O CARDIAC CATH W MCC	6	$22	$2,532	$6,650	$10	$350	$4,978	$11,987	$3,555	$796	$636	$214	$31,730	45.9	
236	CORONARY BYPASS W/O CARDIAC CATH W/O MCC	41	$0	$1,184	$3,221	$124	$240	$1,651	$11,195	$1,834	$335	$370	$123	$20,277	31.9	

Note: Shaded areas represent components that exceed benchmark cost per case. DRG = diagnosis-related group; LOS = length of stay; med–surg = medical and surgical nursing unit.

- Provider
- Process
- Population

Each level is discussed in detail in the following paragraphs.

Utilization Improvement at the Component Level

A component-level benchmarking analysis reveals functional services with cost and utilization rates that exceed those of other organizations. High component costs often reflect high rates of service utilization, but they may also reflect productivity, supply, or other operational challenges. For example, a high nursing cost per case could be an artifact of high LOS, an inefficient nurse staffing model, or both issues. In these instances, cross-referencing clinical benchmarking with productivity and other measures is important to differentiate utilization opportunities from other issues.

Using the following strategies, improvement teams should identify component-level interventions that lower costs across multiple patient populations:

- Review inpatient nursing care team staffing, and develop new models to reduce labor expense per patient day.
- Identify overutilization of ancillary testing and therapies, particularly when demand is driven by standard order sets. Particular focus should be on
  - laboratory services,
  - medical imaging,
  - physical and occupational therapy,
  - respiratory therapy, and
  - noninvasive cardiac testing.
- Identify opportunities to reduce pharmaceutical expenses, particularly with the use of
  - antibiotics,

- antivirals,
- antineoplastics,
- antihyperlipidemics,
- ulcer drugs, and
- antiarthritics.
- Reduce costs of cardiac, orthopedic, and spine implants through
  - improved pricing,
  - demand matching, and
  - stent procedure management.
- Reduce labor-related expenses in perioperative services through
  - team design,
  - block scheduling,
  - throughput enhancements,
  - case length management, and
  - intraoperative monitoring.

Utilization Improvement at the Diagnosis Level

DRG-level clinical benchmarking can reveal utilization and cost improvement opportunities at the diagnosis and service line levels. High-volume, highly complex DRGs drive a majority of inpatient expenses and often experience significant variation in utilization across providers. These DRG areas are often the best candidates for acute care clinical improvement teams to take on. Exhibit 8.6 shows a list of 15 DRGs that are common sources for utilization improvement for most hospitals.

Each DRG presents unique opportunities that can be anticipated by team leaders. For example, a team that works on cardiac stent case costs can expect to find the most opportunities in the following areas:

- Nursing critical care utilization
- Blood conservation

- Surgery case length
- Stent utilization and demand matching
- Laboratory test utilization
- Pharmacy utilization

In contrast, case costs for septicemia and other general medicine procedures are often driven by LOS, use of ICU services, and pharmaceutical expenses.

Exhibit 8.6: Top 15 Clinical Utilization Improvement Areas

Service Line	Diagnoses	MS-DRGs
Cardiology	Cardiac valve replacement	216, 217, 219, 220, 221
	Heart failure	291, 292, 293
	Cardiac stents	246, 247, 248, 249
	Cardiac pacemaker	242, 243, 244
	AMI	280, 281, 282, 283, 284, 285
Orthopedics	Joint replacement	470
Neonatology	Neonate with major problem	792, 793, 794
General medicine	Septicemia	870, 871, 872
	Pneumonia	193, 194, 195
	Infectious disease with OR procedure	853, 854, 855
Neurosurgery	Craniotomy	24, 25, 26, 27
	Spinal fusion	459, 460, 471, 472, 473
General surgery	Small and large bowel procedures	329, 330, 331
Gastroenterology	Esophagitis	391, 392
Dermatology	Cellulitis	602, 603

Source: Based on Galloway Consulting's collective experience across numerous clients.

Note: AMI = acute myocardial infarction; MS-DRG = Medicare-severity diagnosis-related group; OR = operating room.

Utilization Improvement at the Provider Level

Cost-per-case analysis can reveal extensive performance variation among physicians for similar patient types. Collaborative teams need to identify outlier physicians whose costs per case offer improvement opportunities. In these cases, the improvement intervention may focus on one or two physicians rather than involving the full group or specialty.

Exhibit 8.7 is a cost-per-case analysis by physician for craniotomy procedures associated with trauma cases. The data are based on an all-patient refined DRG methodology, which accounts for acuity levels in a DRG (AHRQ 2017). As shown in the exhibit, physician C has the highest volume of cases as well as the highest cost per case of his peer surgeons, exceeding the breakeven cost per case determined by the organization. To improve his performance, a collaborative team should work with physician C to improve rather than engaging all the surgeons in the PI initiative.

Exhibit 8.7: Example of Physician Cost per Case Variation for Procedure Code APR 20, Craniotomy for Trauma (Level 3)

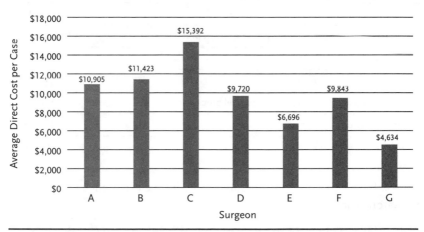

Utilization Improvement at the Process Level

Health systems need effective processes, including throughput efficiency measures, to ensure that patients are placed in the care environment that best meets their medical needs. For example, hospitals must rely on expedient processes to transition patients from acute care to long-term care, home health, and other post-acute services. Poor transfer protocols and processes delay discharges and increase LOS for many patients.

Excessive utilization can be the result of inefficient or ineffective clinical or support processes and systems. Improving these processes can result in utilization improvements that lower operating expenses. For example, LOS improvement can reduce staffing requirements on inpatient units and lower routine care and testing for laboratory, imaging, pharmacy, rehabilitation services, and other clinical services.

Prior to launching clinical improvement teams, the organization should conduct an analysis of inpatient LOS performance. Typically, LOS is compared by case and by DRG to the Medicare geometric mean LOS (or other proprietary benchmarks), and a total "excess days" count (the number of days that exceed the geometric mean) is determined by diagnosis and service line (exhibit 8.8). LOS reduction can be employed as a key improvement strategy, particularly with nonsurgical DRGs in which costs are highly correlated with the number of patient days accrued.

In addition to calculating averages by DRG, organizations may drill down in a diagnosis to gauge the impact of outlier cases on the average. When possible, organizations should also evaluate LOS by nursing service component, such as critical care, step-down unit, and routine nursing. This assessment enables leaders to identify the occurrence of critical care overutilization. Transferring less acute patients to a step-down unit can lower the costs of care by avoiding high-cost critical care services.

Exhibit 8.8: Analysis of Excess Days (partial list)

DRG	DRG Description	Total Cases	Transfer DRG?	CMS Geometric Mean	Avg LOS	Total Excess Days	Positive Excess Days	Negative Excess Days	Positive Days Per Case
386	EXTREME IMMATURITY OR RESPIRATORY DISTRESS SYNDROME, NEONATE	35	No	17.9	36.3	643	751	(109)	21.5
576	SEPTICEMIA W/O MV96+ HOURS AGE >17	292	Yes	5.5	5.6	42	450	(408)	1.5
541	ECMO OR TRACH W MV 96+HRS OR PDX EXC FACE, MOUTH & NECK W MAJ O.R.	20	Yes	37.0	53.9	337	419	(82)	21.0
373	VAGINAL DELIVERY W/O COMPLICATING DIAGNOSES	1,324	No	2.1	2.1	33	375	(342)	0.3
461	O.R. PROC W DIAGNOSES OF OTHER CONTACT W HEALTH SERVICES	16	No	3.3	26.0	363	372	(8)	23.2
316	RENAL FAILURE	263	Yes	4.8	4.8	1	338	(337)	1.3
127	HEART FAILURE & SHOCK	294	Yes	4.1	4.1	13	334	(321)	1.1
578	INFECTIOUS & PARASITIC DISEASES W OR PROCEDURE	52	Yes	12.7	15.2	129	284	(156)	5.5
87	PULMONARY EDEMA & RESPIRATORY FAILURE	122	No	4.9	5.8	106	249	(142)	2.0
75	MAJOR CHEST PROCEDURES	81	Yes	7.4	8.9	125	239	(115)	3.0
544	MAJOR JOINT REPLACEMENT OR REATTACHMENT OF LOWER EXTREMITY	509	Yes	4.0	3.7	(154)	207	(361)	0.4

(continued)

(continued from previous page)

Exhibit 8.8: Analysis of Excess Days (partial list)

DRG	DRG Description	Total Cases	Transfer DRG?	CMS Geometric Mean	Avg LOS	Total Excess Days	Positive Excess Days	Negative Excess Days	Positive Days Per Case
14	INTRACRANIAL HEMORRHAGE OR CEREBRAL INFARCTION	166	Yes	4.3	4.2	(14)	205	(218)	1.2
385	NEONATES, DIED OR TRANSFERRED TO ANOTHER ACUTE CARE FACILITY	23	No	1.8	9.6	179	188	(10)	8.2
188	OTHER DIGESTIVE SYSTEM DIAGNOSES AGE >17 W CC	83	Yes	4.0	5.2	101	187	(86)	2.3
138	CARDIAC ARRHYTHMIA & CONDUCTION DISORDERS W CC	193	No	3.0	3.1	26	178	(152)	0.9
371	CESAREAN SECTION W/O CC	493	No	3.1	3.2	39	164	(126)	0.3
88	CHRONIC OBSTRUCTIVE PULMONARY DISEASE	163	No	4.0	3.9	(15)	163	(178)	1.0
210	HIP & FEMUR PROCEDURES EXCEPT MAJOR JOINT AGE >17 W CC	77	Yes	5.9	7.1	92	159	(67)	2.1

Note: Data are ranked by positive excess days according to diagnosis-related group (DRG). CMS = Centers for Medicare & Medicaid Services; LOS = length of stay.

Utilization Improvement at the Population Level

Health systems have begun to participate in risk-based programs to manage the overall health of defined populations. The goals of these programs are to reduce costs and improve clinical outcomes by managing the totality of a patient's healthcare utilization in all its aspects: experiences of care, health status, and the per capita costs of care (Berwick, Nolan, and Whittington 2008).

Population health management mandates will eventually require organizations to evaluate total medical services across defined cohort groups. To manage population health effectively, health systems need access to, and the ability to analyze, encounter-level data on medical service utilization. Consider the example of a multispecialty physician group that is contracted with two commercial health plans to provide primary and specialty care on a fixed revenue per member per month basis. The group sought to measure and improve specialty drug utilization and expense for populations for both plans. Using claims data, the group evaluated prescription rates and costs by drug and identified the costliest products. Exhibit 8.9 shows the pharmaceutical units dispensed per 1,000 members per month for the populations' top 20 specialty drugs.

The analysis shows the variation in units and daily consumption by drug for the two plans. The medical group compared these rates to external benchmarks to identify drugs that are over- and under-prescribed. This work was extended to the provider level to evaluate prescribing practices by physician. Additionally, the group evaluated usage per member cohort of each drug to understand how medications were administered for specific medical conditions.

Clinical collaborative teams are instrumental in helping drive utilization improvement in health systems. The following is a case example of a clinical team charged with lowering costs and improving margins on high-volume inpatient services. The case illustrates the interplay of operational and utilization improvement that both helped lower case costs.

CASE EXAMPLE: CLINICAL UTILIZATION IMPROVEMENT TEAM

At a large teaching hospital, a multidisciplinary team of physicians and clinicians was charged with identifying annual savings opportunities of $5 million to $7.5 million in inpatient clinical utilization. The team, under the executive leadership of the chief nursing officer and the CMO, met over a seven-week period using a rapid-cycle process, as shown in exhibit 8.10. Core team members included physicians representing each clinical area and representatives from nursing, pharmacy, laboratory, and other clinical service areas.

The first two meetings were spent reviewing DRG-level cost-per-case data and the organization's performance compared with that of other hospital systems. The team's data analyst cross-referenced the clinical benchmark results with productivity benchmark results to discern instances where high case costs were driven by factors other than utilization. For example, a high cost per case in obstetrics was reflective of a low volume of deliveries in labor and delivery.

Most of the analytic and idea-vetting work was conducted between meetings using subteams. These teams were assigned during meeting 2 to address service lines that were shown as promising the most improvement opportunities. The subteams reviewed department-level information and benchmarking results to determine areas where the organization's costs were higher than the benchmarks. Further drill-down to the charge-item level (e.g., pharmacy, imaging, cardiac services) enabled the team to understand the type of services and products that were most overutilized. The teams also researched external, evidence-based care practices to identify clinical improvements and support the continuation of some internal practices.

Beginning in meeting 3, the subteams reported their findings and recommendations to the core team. These ideas were vetted, rated for level of risk, and recorded in a tracking sheet. The data analyst supported the core team in assessing the potential economic opportunities with each identified initiative.

Exhibit 8.9: Per Member per Month (PMPM) Specialty Drug Utilization Analysis (top 20 by total spend)

Drug Name	Drug	Therapeutic Class	Health Plan A				Health Plan B			
			2-Year Spend	No. of Prescriptions for Period	Units/ 1,000 PMPM	DACON	2-Year Spend	No. of Prescriptions for Period	Units/ 1,000 PMPM	DACON
Abilify	A	Antipsychotics/antimanic agents	$2,749,888	3,683	56.29	1.06	$1,897,426	2,161	67.00	1.12
Crestor	B	Antihyperlipidemics	$2,022,266	11,059	173.14	0.99	$1,915,552	8,695	163.14	1.00
Dextroamphet-amine—Amphet ER	C	ADHD/antinarcolepsy/antiobesity/anorexiants	$2,034,059	12,243	215.49	1.27	$1,042,548	6,691	236.09	1.27
Advair diskus	D	Antiasthmatic and bronchodilator agents	$1,052,139	3,890	113.05	1.99	$1,455,892	4,446	214.59	2.00
Humalog	E	Antidiabetics	$1,382,294	3,410	36.67	0.70	$1,031,104	2,169	35.93	0.74
Oxycontin	F	Analgesics—opioid	$1,485,813	2,863	100.39	2.74	$725,994	1,533	85.58	2.44
Suboxone	G	Analgesics—opioid	$1,390,959	5,164	99.76	1.94	$816,950	2,866	47.79	1.83
Lantus Solostar	H	Antidiabetics	$1,200,664	3,397	30.66	0.55	$902,480	2,331	35.42	0.59
Proair HFA	I	Antiasthmatic and bronchodilator agents	$1,127,161	24,033	102.08	0.39	$636,317	12,012	108.26	0.42
Atorvastatin calcium	J	Antihyperlipidemics	$1,371,234	33,846	547.75	1.00	$330,645	22,757	711.03	1.00
Methylphenidate ER	K	ADHD/antinarcolepsy/antiobesity/anorexiants	$1,101,028	6,741	113.88	1.20	$578,637	3,395	146.62	1.19
Flovent HFA	L	Antiasthmatic and bronchodilator agents	$919,753	5,463	30.34	0.38	$605,223	3,038	46.83	0.39

(continued)

(continued from previous page)

Exhibit 8.9: Per Member per Month (PMPM) Specialty Drug Utilization Analysis (top 20 by total spend)

Drug Name	Drug	Therapeutic Class	Health Plan A				Health Plan B			
			2-Year Spend	No. of Prescriptions for Period	Units/ 1,000 PMPM	DACON	2-Year Spend	No. of Prescriptions for Period	Units/ 1,000 PMPM	DACON
Viagra	M	Cardiovascular agents—miscellaneous	$829,971	7,833	15.16	0.19	$680,733	5,634	20.49	0.15
Amphetamine salt combo	N	ADHD/antinarcolepsy/antiobesity/anorexiants	$794,297	12,027	334.88	2.02	$486,786	7,046	399.56	2.01
Fluticasone propionate	O	Dermatologicals	$1,009,691	29,642	234.50	0.55	$217,321	13,616	246.08	0.56
Januvia	P	Antidiabetics	$981,550	3,314	54.46	1.02	$244,111	688	35.14	1.04
Modafinil	Q	ADHD/antinarcolepsy/antiobesity/anorexiants	$966,440	1,126	27.82	1.65	$247,733	254	22.69	1.46
Epipen 2-Pak	R	Vasosuppressors	$806,633	2,740	2.79	0.29	$374,818	1,070	3.84	0.28
Onetouch Ultra test strips	S	Diagnostic products	$862,176	5,875	357.73	3.88	$109,425	309	543.25	7.38
Harvoni	T	Antivirals	$776,955	24	0.31	1.00	$188,244	6	0.07	1.00
			$24,864,971				$14,487,938			

Note: ADHD = attention deficit hyperactivity disorder; DACON = daily average consumption; ER = extended release.

Exhibit 8.10: Clinical Improvement Team Recommendations (partial list)

Meeting 1	• Educate core team on process and charter. • Review initial benchmark analysis; identify improvement opportunities for key sub–service lines. • Cross-reference cost-per-case variances with productivity performance to discern utilization opportunities. • Review cost of off-quality and value-based purchasing benchmark data.
Between meetings	• Complete remaining benchmarking analytics. • Develop analytic template for top sub–service line opportunity (cost per case, length of stay, opportunity matrix).
Meeting 2	• Finalize prioritized list of 10–15 sub–service lines; charter subteams. • Work through detailed example of top sub–service line; identify initial improvement opportunities. • Review detailed clinical benchmarking data.
Between meetings	• Document and size initial opportunities identified in meeting 2. • Prepare analytics for next 3–4 sub–service lines.
Meeting 3	• Finalize sizing of opportunities from previous meeting. • Work through detail of next 3–4 sub–service lines. • Identify improvement opportunities.
Between meetings	• Document and size initial opportunities identified in meeting 3. • Prepare analytics for next 3–4 sub–service lines. • Launch inquiries into opportunities with other benchmark organizations.
Meeting 4	• Finalize sizing of opportunities from previous meeting. • Work through detail of next 3–4 sub–service lines. • Identify improvement opportunities.
Between meetings	• Document and size initial opportunities identified in meeting 4. • Prepare analytics for next 3–4 sub–service lines. • Schedule and meet with physicians to review and vet opportunities.
Meeting 5	• Complete review of remaining sub–service lines. • Discuss opportunities identified via external benchmarking. • Discuss input from physician meetings.
Between meetings	• Document and size opportunities identified in meeting 5. • Schedule and meet with remaining physicians to review and vet opportunities.
Meeting 6	• Finalize risk ratings and sizing of opportunities. • Begin drafting implementation plan. • Finalize communication plan.
Between meetings	• Work toward completion of implementation plan. • Draft communication plan.
Meeting 7	• Finalize implementation plan. • Finalize communication plan. • Prepare for communication to steering committee.

Most of the opportunity was found to reside in ten primary sub–service lines:

- Neonates with major problems
- Tracheostomy
- Cardiac surgery
- Infectious diseases
- Pulmonology
- General surgery
- Gastroenterology
- Spine fusions
- Craniotomy
- Deliveries

At the conclusion of the seven weeks, the team had identified 55 improvement opportunities totaling $5.1 million in risk-rated annual cost improvement opportunity. The recommendations covered numerous service areas and issues, as shown in exhibit 8.11.

The team learned that cost per case performance is driven by more than utilization. Other factors, such as staffing models, supply chain factors, and other operational components, are often key drivers of cost per case. Consequently, the team's recommendations included operational improvements, particularly in staffing models on the patient care units and in surgery.

The combined savings represented an improvement of 12 to 20 percent of a DRG's expense base, depending on the service line. This information was presented to the steering leadership team assigned to oversee the clinical teams. Once the steering team approved the recommendations, the team developed a detailed implementation plan to assign responsibilities and timing.

Exhibit 8.11: Clinical Improvement Team Recommendations (partial list)

Sub–Service Line	Recommended Improvement Areas
Neonates with major problem	NICU care model, LOS, laboratory, respiratory, imaging, TPN usage, nitric oxygen usage
Cardiac valves	CVICU care model, LOS (ICU and overall), surgery expense, cardiac testing
Cardiac—CABG	CVICU care model, lab and pharmacy utilization, blood utilization
Septicemia	LOS (ICU and overall), lab and imaging utilization
Spinal fusions	Intraoperative monitoring usage, surgery supplies, biologic usage, LOS
Pneumonia	LOS, lab and pharmacy utilization, vent management

Note: CABG = coronary artery bypass graft; CVICU = cardiovascular intensive care unit; ICU = intensive care unit; LOS = length of stay; NICU = neonatal intensive care unit; TPN = total parenteral nutrition.

CHAPTER 9

Building Revenues

THE PERFORMANCE IMPROVEMENT (PI) levers presented to this point address process and operational cost improvement opportunities. Although cost management is a vital component of organizational performance, it cannot be the sole source of improvement. Health systems cannot solely focus on expense reduction and expect to survive over the long term. Hospitals are largely fixed-cost operations and, as such, must generate sufficient volumes and revenues to cover overhead expenses. For this reason, PI must include component initiatives to drive growth in market share and optimize net revenues and contribution margins.

While the need for revenue growth is self-evident, developing and executing effective growth strategies for health systems is challenging. Most health systems face increased competition for a shrinking acute care market. Furthermore, competition is growing in the outpatient services market segment, fueled in part by the emergence of nontraditional service providers such as retail pharmacies offering on-site primary care physician services.

Revenue growth is not simply aimed at increasing patient volumes. The higher patient volumes must occur in conjunction with growth in revenues and contribution margins to cover operating expenses. Growth in low-margin services or payer groups can erode the organization's operating margins. Providers must effectively compete for high-margin, commercially insured patients while streamlining costs to improve Medicare and Medicaid margin performance.

Growth strategies also must shift with the ever-changing complexities of healthcare reimbursement. With the advent of population health management, providers are paid increasingly on an at-risk basis. To remain viable, health systems will seek to grow revenues through managing the health of defined patient populations. Under these arrangements, providers are at risk to reduce unnecessary utilization to maintain margins. In contrast to fee-for-service, value-based reimbursement reduces patient volumes for some services and increases demand for others.

Exhibit 9.1 contrasts some of the margin strategies under fee-for-service and population health reimbursement. In most cases, provider incentives under population health are antithetical to fee-for-service.

Exhibit 9.1: Margin Tactics—Fee-for-Service Versus Population Health

Margin Tactics—Fee-for-Service		Margin Tactics—Population Health
Increase inpatient volumes.	➡	Decrease inpatient volumes.
Increase diagnostic procedure volumes.	➡	Decrease diagnostic testing.
Focus on specialty care.	➡	Focus on primary care.
Invest capital in facilities, equipment.	➡	Invest capital in systems and services to monitor and "pull" patients early in disease state.

As the industry transitions to population health, providers must determine how to work in both worlds.

HIGH-GROWTH HEALTH SYSTEMS

High-performing health systems are adept at sustaining revenues and market share growth. Some systems are fortunate to serve growing markets and patients with favorable insurance coverage. Other organizations achieve growth despite entrenched competition and similar market challenges.

High-growth healthcare organizations have competencies in the areas discussed in this section.

Portfolio Management

High-growth healthcare systems employ the principles of portfolio management. These organizations judiciously apply the required levels of capital investment to grow programs and generate operating margins necessary for reinvestment. High-growth organizations create a strategic advantage in key, high-margin services and are willing to restructure, outsource, or eliminate underperforming programs. Executives pursue selective acquisitions to grow market share, strengthen business portfolios, and improve service delivery to the communities served.

Reputation for Clinical Quality

Patients, physicians, payers, and employers are drawn to provider organizations with a reputation for providing high-quality healthcare. The publication of quality data further molds consumers' perceptions and purchasing decisions. Conversely, organizations with a reputation of providing low-quality care will encounter increasing difficulty in growing service demand.

Reputation for Service Quality

High-growth healthcare organizations excel at customer service and enjoy high patient satisfaction survey scores. They achieve this reputation by fostering an organizational culture committed to continuously improving services provided to patients and families. The organization aligns the workforce with service goals and provides the tools and training to deliver customer-responsive service.

Capacity and Access

Health systems must have sufficient service capacity to accommodate growing caseloads. Facilities and programs that operate at full capacity restrict access for patients and frustrate physicians. Organizations that excel in capacity management take the following steps:

- Schedule patient appointments, tests, and procedures in a timely manner.
- Consistently maintain capacity in surgery to accommodate additional cases.
- Minimize emergency department (ED) diversions caused by inpatient bed shortages.
- Minimize patient waiting times in physician offices, the ED, and other ambulatory care settings.
- Locate services in the market to ensure convenience and access for patients.
- Provide convenient parking and effective signage and other wayfinding information to assist patients and families.

Physician Alignment

High-growth healthcare organizations are aligned with their affiliated physicians and work collaboratively with them to pursue market and growth opportunities. These organizations avoid competition with physicians and seek joint ventures and other arrangements to align caregivers and share in revenue growth.

Referral Network Management

High-growth providers are effective at attracting and retaining new patients. When these patients require a referral, the organization is adept at steering most of these cases to an affiliated provider. Competency in referral management reflects the following attributes:

- The organization is effective at identifying and retaining new patients.
- The organization focuses attention and support on providers who offer clinical leadership and loyalty to the organization.
- The health system has processes in place that make referrals seamless and easy for referring physicians and other providers to use.
- The organization tracks referrals to specialty services and for acute care admissions and minimizes leakage of cases to competitors.

Sales Competency

Healthcare organizations are big businesses and require competencies in sales and marketing that are commonly found in other industries. High-growth organizations develop sales and marketing approaches to attract and retain patients and physicians. Effective referral tracking and management minimize the loss of patients and business to competitors. For health systems, sales competencies are evident when

- dedicated staff and resources are assigned to market to and build relationships with physicians, health plans, employer groups, and other external targets;
- business development staff are equipped with customer relationship management (CRM) tools and other systems to manage sales execution;
- pay incentives are in place for staff who have growth responsibilities;
- the organization has invested in business intelligence to build understanding of the local healthcare market and to support investments and service expansion;
- marketing resources and promotional campaigns are aligned to support growth strategies and to build brand awareness and market share; and
- the organization has cultivated deep expertise to support effective pricing and negotiation practices with payers.

LEVER 14: DEMAND GROWTH

Growth-focused collaborative teams should be a component of most organizational transformation and improvement projects. The scope of a growth team can vary depending on the size of the organization and the potential for growth. Targets for growth teams are generally stated in terms of increased net patient revenues, but they may also be stated as a percentage of growth in cases, visits, or procedures.

As shown in exhibit 9.2, a growth team can focus simultaneously on several programs and service lines. Frequently, these areas are assigned to separate subteams.

The chief strategy officer or CEO typically serves as the executive sponsor, while the top executive for planning and marketing

Exhibit 9.2: Example of a Growth Collaborative Team Structure

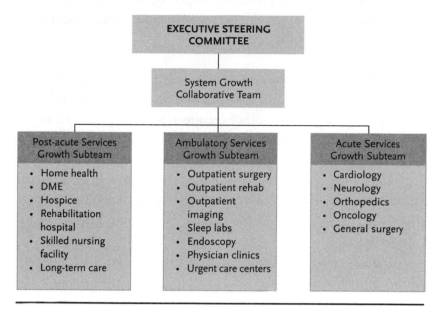

Note: DME = durable medical equipment.

is the team leader. Selection of members depends on the scope of the team's work; however, membership typically includes program and service line directors, business development and finance staff, physician liaisons, and decision support analysts.

Growth teams require information to measure current program performance and identify market opportunities, including the following:

- Current patient volumes and trends to identify capacity issues and understand which programs are growing or declining
- Service line profit and loss information to understand programmatic margin performance
- Market data to foresee the potential for growth in the service area

- Data on referrals to measure provider productivity and the prevalence of cases sent to competing organizations
- Data on other provider organizations to understand the competitive landscape

Growth-oriented teams typically focus on short-term tactical opportunities, structural improvements to systems and staff that support growth and sales execution, and long-term strategic growth initiatives to increase patient volumes and revenues (exhibit 9.3). High-performing health systems build a culture and set of disciplines that emphasize a continuous focus on strategic growth. Such a culture can only emerge through leadership and physician alignment, data-driven decision making, and strong core operating competencies.

Tactical growth can occur when some or all of the following approaches are employed:

- Working with community physicians who send cases to competing organizations (e.g., "splitters") to bring more business to the health system
- Addressing process and system issues that prevent physicians from sending more business to the organization
- Reducing leakage of referrals, particularly from owned physician practices
- Creating new demand and revenues through diligent documentation of patient conditions and referrals to the appropriate specialty service or clinician
- Freeing capacity in surgery and other outpatient departments to reduce case backlogs
- Redeploying providers and resources to new care sites to build capacity in growing markets

Strategic growth strategies take longer than tactical growth initiatives to yield results, but they may be included in the scope of a

Exhibit 9.3: Dimensions of Health System Growth

Increasing Depth ↑	Tactical	Structural	Strategic
Intrinsic and Substantive (lifestyle)	**"A single root cause will fix our problems":** • Growth initiatives are data driven. • Understanding of the performance of core competencies driving growth is evident. • Efforts are isolated, bottom-up or top-down activities. • Focus is on tactical approaches, not necessarily tied to core competencies. • Some areas consistently perform better than others. • Growth is a goal for some.	**Focused set of root issue improvements:** • "It's all about physicians and service." • The organizational structure is partially integrated. • Structural solutions are not necessarily driven by strategy (e.g., physician liaison). • Some efforts are seen to transfer "successes" across organization.	**Deep and broad change for all:** • Integrated growth plans are instituted. • All core competencies show strength. • Core competency improvements are linked. • All senior leaders are very committed. • Everyone is involved; change is systemic. • Employees are empowered.
Superficial and Mechanical (diet)	**No comprehensive plan:** • "It's all about marketing and promotion." • Projects are reactive. • Priorities are based on instinct and intuitive knowledge. • Growth initiatives do not get prioritized. • Individual leaders select growth priorities.	**Focused department/function:** • Some senior leaders support improvement across departments. • Overarching belief is that the issues are about both people and processes. • Specific roles/functions are redesigned; a few departments own improvement. • Concern is felt that a focus on patient satisfaction will cost "too much."	**It's about "most" of us:** • Several departments work together. • Some senior leaders own improvement such that they are important to the organization. • Growth plans are not integrated with others as strategic goals. • Growth plans may not address root causes. • Initiatives are sustained through intense focus and effort.

Increasingly Integrated into Culture →

growth-focused collaborative team. Examples of long-term growth initiatives include the following:

- Recruiting physicians toward increasing patient visits, referrals, and procedures
- Developing new systems and support services to link currently unaffiliated community physician practices with the organization
- Investing in existing service lines to increase access and market visibility
- Building programs and care sites through which to pursue additional markets
- Purchasing provider programs to garner market share and market presence
- Launching joint ventures with physicians (e.g., comanagement agreements) and other provider organizations
- Pursuing contracting agreements with payers and employer groups to build volumes and improve reimbursement levels

A growth-focused collaborative team may also assess and improve processes and systems that support growth and sales. For example, a team may take the following steps:

- Evaluate the organization's existing sales organization and recommend improvements concerning roles, structure, and strategies.
- Conduct sales training to build staff proficiencies and effectiveness.
- Implement CRM systems and other tools to support sales and marketing and to track, by provider,
  - inpatient referral volumes, both internal and external;
  - internal outpatient referral volume;
  - service issues and actions; and
  - recent activity with physicians.

- Evaluate and reset priorities for marketing and advertising investments to support growth programs.

Growth teams typically continue intact through the implementation phase of PI to serve as a guiding presence. Sales execution requires significant oversight and tracking. For example, the team should track sales initiatives involving physician meetings and capture the key issues and opportunities that arise from these dialogues. A forum should be provided for sales staff to share lessons and market intelligence that arise during implementation. Consistent oversight also enforces accountability and guidance when implementation plans require modification.

The next case example profiles a subteam focused on growing home health volumes and revenues. It demonstrates the complexities of growing post-acute services and the challenge inherent in marketing to multiple customer groups (i.e., physicians, patients, other facilities).

CASE EXAMPLE: GROWING HOME HEALTH SERVICES

A home health program director was asked to lead a growth-oriented collaborative team. The team was charged with increasing home health and durable medical equipment referrals. The agency was part of a five-hospital system located in a large, competitive metropolitan area. The system's inpatients provided most of the referrals to the agency, but with stagnant growth in inpatient discharges, the home agency was experiencing anemic growth and increased competition from competitor agencies.

As a starting point, the team reviewed six months of home health referral data on Medicare cases from each system hospital. The team discovered that the percentage of Medicare cases referred to the system's home care services varied from 58 percent to 27 percent, with a weighted average of 40 percent (exhibit 9.4). The remaining 60 percent of cases were referred by competing agencies.

The differences by facility were caused in part by the prevalence of competing home care providers in the local area. However, other controllable factors accounted for low percentages for several facilities, including

- preferences in home care services for some discharging physicians,
- preferences and negative perceptions of facility case managers about the system's home health program, and
- differences in how case managers presented the system's home health services as a viable option for patients.

Next, the team conducted a diagnosis-related group (DRG)–level benchmarking analysis (exhibit 9.5) to compare the system's home health disposition rates for Medicare inpatients with regional and national benchmarks. This analysis revealed lower rates than benchmark for several of the system facilities' specialties, including orthopedics, infectious diseases, and cardiology. Additionally, disposition rates varied considerably across providers and case managers.

Exhibit 9.4: Market Share of Internal Home Health Referrals

Referring System Facility	Total Home Health Dispositions for Period (6 months)	System Home Health Dispositions	System Share	Nonsystem Home Health Dispositions
Hospital A	287	166	58%	121
Hospital B	743	377	51%	366
Hospital C	384	149	39%	235
Hospital D	570	178	31%	392
Hospital E	594	161	27%	433
Grand total	**2,578**	**1,031**	**40%**	**1,547**

Exhibit 9.5: Home Health DRG-Level Referrals Analysis Among Medicare Patients

MDC No.	MDC Description	Home Health Referrals	Total Discharges	Percentage of Cases	Percentage			Additional Cases at Benchmark (annualized)		
					Region	State	Top Performers	Region	State	Top Performers
16	Blood diseases and disorders	15	97	15.5%	12.2%	10.7%	30.3%	-6	-9	29
5	Circulatory system	170	1,286	13.2%	15.2%	13.7%	26.4%	52	13	340
6/7	Digestive system, pancreas, and liver	73	582	12.5%	13.1%	11.4%	22.3%	7	-14	114
10	Endocrine, nutritional metabolism	11	81	13.6%	15.2%	13.2%	29.4%	3	-1	26
3	Eye, ear, nose, and throat	3	57	5.3%	10.5%	9.8%	30.0%	6	5	28
18/25	Infectious and parasitic (HIV-AIDS)	18	254	7.1%	12.9%	12.2%	27.3%	30	26	103
11	Kidney and urinary	56	312	17.9%	15.8%	13.9%	26.0%	-13	-25	50
17	Malignancies	1	38	2.6%	18.3%	16.9%	41.7%	12	11	30
19/20	Mental health and substance abuse	2	21	9.5%	2.3%	2.5%	33.3%	-3	-3	10
8	Musculoskeletal system	39	385	10.1%	20.4%	18.5%	36.4%	80	65	203
1	Nervous system	31	321	9.7%	12.0%	10.8%	22.6%	15	7	84
4	Respiratory system	88	497	17.7%	16.1%	13.8%	26.8%	-16	-39	91
9	Skin	21	100	21.0%	20.0%	19.1%	38.1%	-2	-4	34
	Grand Total	**528**	**4,031**	**13.1%**	**15.1%**	**13.5%**	**27.2%**	**162**	**31**	**1,141**

Note: MDC = major diagnostic category.

At the time, 13.1 percent of Medicare discharges were assigned a home health disposition code. If the system performed at regional averages (on the basis of the system's DRG mix and volumes of patients), the revised average would be 16.1 percent. This difference in rates translated to an estimated loss in net revenues of $600,000 per year.

On the basis of these findings, the team identified improvement opportunities to grow referrals through three avenues:

- Increase the percentage of system inpatients referred to the system's home health program. The team developed specific recommendations related to
  - role design and sales training for home health liaisons, sales executives, the home health educator, and intake staff to improve service to physicians, patients, and other facility case managers;
  - collaboration with the organization's internal case managers;
  - implementation of Medicare-compliant scripting for case managers to facilitate their meetings with patients and families; and
  - engagement of the top 15 physicians referring a high percentage of patients outside the system.
- Improve the identification of acute care cases that qualify for home health services by
  - focusing on top-volume DRGs with disposition and referral rates that were lower than regional and national benchmark rates and
  - presenting data to physicians and case managers to identify patient groups that could benefit from home health but are not being referred.
- Increase the market share of home health referrals from other health systems.

From these recommendations, the group further identified opportunities to grow Medicare home health referrals. By working with providers and case managers, the number of cases grew by 15 percent within four months of implementation.

GROWTH AS A PRODUCTIVITY LEVER

Maintaining high labor productivity is easier to accomplish in growing organizations than in those with decreasing patient volumes. The addition of patients produces higher volumes of procedures, tests, and cases, resulting in higher staff utilization. Assuming that growth occurs in populations that feature a favorable payer mix, programs and services that are poised for growth improve productivity and contribution margins by accommodating workload volumes while avoiding or minimizing staffing increases.

Growth revenue targets are typically based on current net revenue margins. Often, growth can be accommodated with existing staff and other resources. When assessing these opportunities for volume, collaborative teams should account for the additional margin generated by the gain in productivity.

LEVER 15: REVENUE OPTIMIZATION

The goal of revenue cycle management for a healthcare organization is to collect the appropriate, optimal cash amount for patient services provided. The net revenue that an organization derives from patient services depends on myriad factors, including the contracts it enters into with payers, how well it enforces compliance with those contracts, and how effectively staff capture, bill, and collect charges.

Revenue cycle management is complex, dynamic, and challenging for most health systems. Arcane reimbursement rules are imposed by third-party payers and can vary widely, creating a complicated system characterized by potential compliance problems, slow cash receipts, and denied or reduced payment of claims. The complexity hinders training of frontline staff in how much to charge for services, what amount to bill for payment, and what amount to accept as full payment.

Reimbursement levels from commercial and governmental payers remain stagnant or are in decline. At the same time, the cost to collect is increasing because of lags in payment, often associated with the increase in out-of-pocket costs for patients enrolled in high-deductible health plans.

High-performing health systems have standard processes and disciplines in place throughout the revenue cycle that reduce variation and lower collection costs. Such effective systems transcend organizational silos and facilitate communication and accountability.

Successful revenue cycle management requires the close collaboration of financial staff and clinicians. Physicians and other clinical staff must provide timely and complete documentation on the patient's condition, diagnoses, and services performed. Department staff must be diligent in charge capture.

Revenue cycle management requires a well-trained, multidisciplinary workforce with proficiencies in payer contracting, coding, claims processing, and many other areas. Billing issues are often a major source of patient dissatisfaction. When interacting with patients, associates must be helpful and knowledgeable.

Staff must be supported by effective, integrated information systems to manage each step of the billing process. Revenue cycle leaders need real-time performance data to measure productivity and track work in process associated with denials; discharged, not final billed (DNFB) accounts; and other patient billing issues.

Revenue cycle management requires the active engagement of patients in the process. Most patients lack clarity on insurance coverage, out-of-pocket expenditures, authorization requirements, eligibility for financial assistance, and other factors. Effective revenue cycle leaders engage patients early in the process, ultimately increasing the net revenues collected.

Revenue Cycle Collaborative Teams

Revenue cycle improvements are a common component of organizational PI initiatives. Hospitals and health systems do not collect all the net revenues due them because of operational and process issues regarding insufficient data collection and documentation, coding errors, ineffective receivables management, and many other areas.

Large PI initiatives frequently include collaborative teams focused on revenue cycle issues and opportunities. The chief financial officer often serves as the executive sponsor, while the team leader may be the organization's vice president of revenue cycle, controller, or patient accounts lead. Selection of members depends on the scope of the initiative, but members typically include representatives from patient accounts, medical records, patient access, clinical documentation improvement, and utilization review.

A revenue cycle team is usually assigned an economic target stated in terms of increased net patient revenues. Revenue cycle targets are often determined by the extent of the gap to be reduced between actual revenues and optimal revenues. For health systems, optimal revenues are the net collections that are possible if the revenue cycle is maximized (e.g., payers are fully compliant with contracts, the organization experiences few denials, claims are submitted without delay). Additional targets may focus on reducing denials, lowering days in accounts receivable, increasing point-of-service (POS) collection rates, and reducing bad debt and other write-offs.

Revenue cycle teams typically perform the following functions:

- Assess current revenue cycle components, and compare them with high-performing industry practices.
- Identify areas of risk and vulnerability in financial reporting and reserve calculations.
- Assess potential risks and opportunities in the areas of receivables and aging accounts, charge capture, billing, and collections.

- Identify needed technology, staff training, and other investments to improve performance and workflow management.

The Health System Revenue Cycle

System gaps at any stage of the revenue process can result in increased denials, increased receivable days, and lowered net revenues. Revenue cycle collaborative teams must assess critical points of the process to identify performance gaps.

Exhibit 9.6 is a high-level depiction of the revenue cycle for health systems. Revenue cycle effectiveness greatly depends on what work has occurred before patient services are provided. Failure to adequately render preservice processes reduces the percentage of clean claims initially submitted, resulting in payment delays and rework. Ideally, all nonemergent patients should have obtained financial clearance, or application for Medicaid or other public assistance, and authorization prior to their admission or outpatient service.

Contracting and Preservice Processes

Many activities in the revenue cycle occur before patients receive medical care. In the first phase of the cycle, organizations seek to verify insurance coverage for patients, secure required authorizations from payers, and collect any out-of-pocket expenses from the patient.

Contracting

Most patients are covered by commercial insurance plans or by Medicare, Medicaid, or another government-sponsored program. Health systems negotiate managed care contracts with commercial insurance companies to provide medical services to enrollees over a defined period. The terms and conditions of these contracts dictate a payer group's reimbursement rates to the organization.

Exhibit 9.6: Health System Revenue Cycle

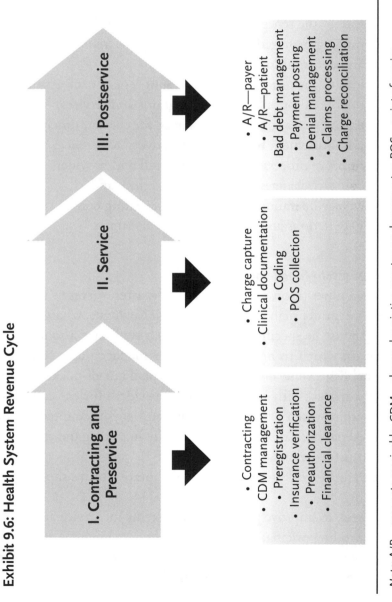

I. Contracting and Preservice	II. Service	III. Postservice
• Contracting	• Charge capture	• A/R—payer
• CDM management	• Clinical documentation	• A/R—patient
• Preregistration	• Coding	• Bad debt management
• Insurance verification	• POS collection	• Payment posting
• Preauthorization		• Denial management
• Financial clearance		• Claims processing
		• Charge reconciliation

Note: A/R = accounts receivable; CDM = charge description master, or chargemaster; POS = point of service.

Specific to contracting issues, revenue cycle teams should pursue interventions that

- strengthen the position of the organization in contract negotiations using modeling and decision support technologies and expertise;
- lead to the renegotiation of terms and conditions with existing managed care payers to improve reimbursement and contribution margins;
- lead to the negotiation of carve-out service contracts for the organization's primary programs and services;
- ensure payer contract compliance for correct, timely reimbursement by auditing the payers' adherence;
- improve processes for notifying staff and providers of contract changes (e.g., terms and rates); and
- engage operational managers in preparing contract negotiations and assimilating new contracts.

Chargemaster Management

A charge description master, or chargemaster, serves as a health system's central pricing and service listing catalogue. Chargemaster pricing must be specific and clear so that staff have a solid foundation on which to negotiate terms for managed care contracts and establish a value on services that are paid out-of-pocket. Prices should correlate with actual costs and provide sufficient contribution margin—even when they are substantially discounted, as for preferred payers. Considering the increase in pricing transparency, prices must be reasonable and competitive.

In their PI work, revenue cycle collaborative teams should

- seek to improve processes and systems for service and product pricing;
- seek to improve the process and timeliness of chargemaster updates resulting from coding changes;

- audit the chargemaster to ensure that reimbursable services are being charged for;
- bundle or eliminate unused codes to help streamline the charging and billing processes;
- implement modified payment plans specifically for self-pay patients;
- simplify billing statements for clarity; and
- survey competitor pricing levels, particularly in the outpatient segment.

Preregistration and Scheduling

Effective revenue cycle management requires complete patient information (financial and demographic) as early as possible in anticipation of the patient encounter. Incorrect or missing patient information leads to increased denials, receivables, and bad debt.

Preregistration is an important process for setting patient expectations regarding insurance coverage and amounts that patients are required to pay out-of-pocket. Patient satisfaction improves when financial responsibility is clearly communicated and coordinated early on.

Most health systems employ centralized call center staff to preregister elective patient admissions and outpatient visits. These staff members are typically responsible for the following tasks:

- Verifying insurance and determining any coordination of benefits
- Providing the patient with an estimate of his or her financial responsibility
- Initiating the preauthorization process
- Collecting payment prior to the service being provided
- Offering financial counseling and help applying for Medicaid or other public assistance

Frequently, the preregistration function also includes scheduling of the service. Registrars may inform the patient of the appropriate preparation for both the exam and financial clearance. Workflow processes should be automatically initiated from the scheduling event to ensure financial clearance, remind patients of appointments, and notify the relevant departments of the patient's arrival.

Centralized scheduling, combined with insurance verification, enables the organization to estimate time delays for authorization. This process can prevent the scheduling of cases before authorizations are completed. Additionally, centralized scheduling permits registrars to offer patients the earliest appointment time available at the most convenient location.

Regarding preregistration functions, revenue cycle teams should accomplish the following:

- Integrate processes, systems, and roles for patient scheduling and registration to improve proficiency and productivity.
- Improve inbound call center performance to minimize hold times and abandonment rates.
- Maximize the percentage of nonemergent patients who are preregistered.
- Minimize the occurrence of scheduling without physician orders or payer authorization.
- Improve processes for verifying medical necessity at the time of scheduling.
- Augment staff training and technologies to improve data capture and accuracy and enhance patient service.
- Implement systems to track front-end errors and direct correction at the point of error.
- Institute processes to track and manage incomplete registrations and medical necessity issues.

Insurance Verification and Benefits Coordination

A central component of the preregistration process is the verification of a patient's insurance coverage. Many patients are not familiar with the specific terms of their insurance and seek assistance. Educating patients about their insurance coverage helps set expectations downstream with billing and collections for facility and professional (physician) services.

Some patients are covered by more than one insurance plan (e.g., a primary plan and supplemental insurance; an individual policy and a spouse's insurance plan), necessitating the coordination of benefits (COB). Medicare patients, for example, must complete the Medicare Secondary Payer questionnaire, which is used to identify secondary insurance and determine the primary and secondary payer.

Preauthorization

Service authorization is a component of insurance verification. Most nonemergent hospital care requires advance authorization from a patient's insurance company. Inpatient admissions, surgeries, medical imaging procedures, and other ambulatory services require the completion of a preauthorization form. Authorization processes and requirements vary by payer. Health systems must continuously monitor and manage payer changes in authorization requirements.

Because authorization must be secured in advance of service performance, incomplete or missing authorization may result in denial of payment from payers. Delays in authorization frequently lead to delays in care, a significant source of dissatisfaction with patients and physicians.

Verification, COB, and preauthorization processes require effective automation and workflow management. Collaborative teams frequently address information system issues as part of their work to improve preservice processes.

Financial Responsibility and Collection

As part of preregistration, patients must be provided an estimate of their expected out-of-pocket expenses. Patients need to be informed of services that are not covered. Medicare (excluding Medicare Advantage) patients, for example, require administration of advance beneficiary notices, which delineate specific services that will not be covered.

This information, along with copayment and deductibles data, is used to calculate an estimate of the patient's out-of-pocket expenses. This analysis is often supported by automated patient estimator tools. Health systems must collect as much of the patient payment in advance of the service as possible, as collection is more difficult and costly to the organization the later it is attempted. At this time, the registrar should be prepared to offer payment options to patients who cannot pay the complete balance up front.

Financial Counseling

A portion of uninsured patients qualify for Medicaid or other available financial assistance. Health systems should assist patients with determining qualification for these programs. Effective counseling can reduce the number of self-pay cases and result in lowered bad debt and write-offs. Financial assistance staff should be trained to educate and communicate with patients and families in a knowledgeable and compassionate manner.

To improve verification, authorization, and financial clearance functions, revenue cycle teams should

- streamline processes for COB;
- improve the timeliness of authorization submissions to reduce delays in care and rescheduling;
- minimize denials associated with authorization issues;
- improve processes for determining patients' estimated financial responsibility;
- increase preservice collections;
- enable preregistration staff to seek coverage for self-paying and uninsured patients through effective screening, application, and financial counseling; and
- improve patient collections by offering payment and loan options up front.

Revenue Cycle Processes at the Time of Service

The revenue cycle process continues at the time a patient arrives for her medical care. Important elements of this phase of the process are discussed next.

Registration

When patients arrive for any medical service, be it an elective admission, a scheduled physician office visit, an unscheduled outpatient procedure, or an ED visit, they first see a patient access representative for registration. For emergency and unscheduled outpatient cases, preregistration does not take place, so verification and collection must occur when patients arrive. Registrars check in patients and collect insurance, billing, and other finance-related information.

The quality and depth of information gathered during this encounter have significant bearing on the success of billing and collections. Registration errors and omissions can produce delayed or rejected claims. Effective registration services require a well-trained workforce supported by highly functioning information systems and routinized processes.

Point-of-Service Collection

High-deductible plans and copayments require health systems to collect cash at the point of service. The consistent practice of effective POS collections improves an organization's cash flow and reduces bad debt and write-offs. Registration staff should be trained in and comfortable using POS collection procedures.

To enhance the patient registration process, revenue cycle collaborative teams should seek to

- optimize registration staff deployment and scheduling to meet demand for inpatient, outpatient, and ED services such that it is sufficient to meet peak demand and minimize patient waiting time;

- improve the quality of data capture through staff training, improved information systems, and standardized procedures;
- convert as many self-pay outpatient and ED patients as possible through effective screening, clearance, and financial counseling;
- increase POS collections at registration via scripting to support registrars in their dialogue with patients; and
- strengthen processes for posting payments from POS collections.

Charge Capture

All patient service areas, from medical imaging to cardiac services to rehabilitative services to physician offices, must capture and record charge transactions for the products used and services provided. Ineffective charging processes result in lost revenues and delays in billing.

Revenue cycle collaborative teams should evaluate the organization's charge capture issues and develop interventions that accomplish the following:

- Reduce the incidence of lost charges and associated lost net revenue, particularly in surgery, outpatient services, and the ED.
- Leverage technologies (e.g., bar coding, supply kiosks) to automate charge capture for high-cost supplies.
- Reduce delays in charging fees after services are rendered in departments by instituting effective charge audit and reconciliation processes and holding leaders accountable for achieving the expected reduction.
- Implement automated systems for daily charge-capture auditing and for communicating back to departments on issues that disrupt the revenue cycle.

Clinical Documentation and Coding

Health systems bill third-party payers using uniform billing templates. Claims summarize the services performed for patients with each service assigned an industry-uniform code (e.g., Current Procedural Terminology code set). A clean claim requires complete, accurate coding supported by clear clinical documentation, which typically originates in the electronic health record. Accurate documentation is required to capture chargeable elements of the patient's condition and medical care, including the following:

- Patient conditions that are present on admission
- Primary and secondary diagnoses
- Patient severity, comorbidities, and mortality risk
- Incidence of off-quality events

Insufficient documentation and coding is a significant and problematic source of revenue cycle dysfunction, as it can lead to

- delays in billing, or an increased incidence of accounts that are DNFB;
- an under- or overstated case mix index;
- increases in accounts receivable days;
- compliance risks and exposure to recovery audit contractor (RAC) audits; and
- increased billing denials.

Revenue cycle collaborative teams almost always encounter challenges with clinical documentation and coding. Teams should address issues that will increase the rate of clean claims submission and reduce the incidence of denials by taking the following steps:

- Institute a clinical documentation improvement program focused on increased training and support for physicians and other clinicians.

- Improve clinical documentation relating to medical necessity.
- Audit and identify services and diagnoses where assigned coding over- or undercategorizes patient conditions.
- Clearly delineate coding timelines to provide timely billing and avoid write-offs.
- Improve coding quality through staff development and effective software support.
- Reduce compliance risks and the incidence of RAC audits.

Postservice Processes

The remaining component of the revenue cycle occurs after services are rendered and primarily involves billing and collection processes performed by the patient accounting department. Tasks include

- generating and submitting claims to payers,
- managing billing receivables from patients and payers,
- posting payments and updating accounts,
- following up on denials, and
- resolving outstanding debt.

Claims Processing

Patient accounts staff are responsible for generating and submitting claims to insurance companies and other payers. Ideally, clean claims are achieved on the first submission attempt, but internal and external factors often prevent this from occurring.

To address claims processing issues, revenue cycle collaborative teams should seek opportunities to

- reduce the incidence of DNFB accounts;
- maximize the percentage of clean claims on first submission;

- improve processes and timeliness for follow-up on rejected claims;
- reduce the rate of duplicate claims submitted; and
- improve processes and tools for managing claims work queues, workflow, and tracking.

Patient Accounts Receivable

Receivables management processes determine the interval of time the health system receives payment for services rendered. Prolonged accounts receivable (A/R) days negatively affect the organization's cash flow and drive up collections and bad debt accounts.

Collaborative teams should capitalize on A/R improvement opportunities such as the following:

- Improving A/R collectability through standardization and rigorous front-end processes
- Improving systems for managing follow-up with payers and patients
- Grouping work teams around key payers and patient cohorts to improve staff proficiency and expertise
- Improving systems for A/R staff development, productivity management, and accountability

Posting Payments and Updating Accounts

During the period an account is open, health systems receive payments from insurance companies and patients. Patient accounting requires effective systems to post these transactions so that all parties are apprised of the current account status and aware of any remaining balances. Accurate posting is critical for preparing the final bill that reflects a patient payment obligation once all insurance remuneration has been received.

Denials Management

Rejected claims and denials pose a major challenge to most healthcare revenue cycle leaders. Denials are often an artifact of process issues and problems that occur early in the billing cycle. Payment denials increase A/R days and raise the risk of bad debt and write-offs. Revenue cycle leaders should institute the following improvements:

- Fully leverage systems for denials tracking and management.
- Improve process flows and automation for rebilling denials and appeals.
- Evaluate denials by payer, physician, registrar, and diagnosis to identify root causes and improvement opportunities.
- Audit managed care contracts to challenge denials and provide input for use in future contract negotiations.
- Organize and deploy a standing technical team focused on denials and their resolution.

Bad Debt and Account Write-Offs

Revenue cycle executives must seek interventions and process changes to minimize the amount of bad debt and the frequency of accounts that are written off. Collaborative teams should focus on decreasing avoidable write-offs through root cause analysis, denial follow-up, account resolution, and performance improvement. Specifically, they should identify opportunities to

- decrease bad debt write-offs through improved financial clearance, self-pay conversions, and improved patient residual collections;
- improve cash collections through reduced payment variances with aggressive expected payment collection efforts;
- develop and implement an avoidable write-off adjustment policy with appropriate levels of authority; and
- provide a feedback loop for informing line staff about denials or operational write-offs.

Professional Services Billing and the Revenue Cycle

The revenue cycle for physician and professional services has similar issues and challenges to those described thus far. Physician billing and coding systems differ from those of hospital services, however, and therefore require different expertise. Small physician enterprises must rely on practice-level staff and physicians to perform eligibility screening, service authorizations, coding, and records management.

Most health systems that operate a physician enterprise employ billing services and staffing that are separate from the hospital business office. Often, organizations charter collaborative teams that focus on revenue cycle issues specific to physician practices and professional billing.

CHAPTER 10

Optimizing the Service Portfolio

COLLECTIVELY, THE DIVERSE clinical programs and services spanning the continuum of care and medical specialties define a health system's clinical services portfolio. Organizations routinely make programmatic portfolio investment decisions throughout the year and as part of the annual budgeting process.

High-performing healthcare systems are adept at managing their service portfolios. These organizations institute evidence-based practices and disciplines to craft portfolio offerings that evolve with marketplace changes. In particular, the following characterize performance excellence related to the service portfolio:

- An optimal portfolio mix of brand, volume, and margin services is determined and reviewed annually. (*Optimal* is a relative term that takes into consideration the strategic, operating, and mission objectives of the organization.)
- Operating results for each service line, and each service, are evaluated at least annually for effectiveness against the stated expectations of their role in the organization's success model and optimal portfolio.
- Monthly and quarterly measurement of success against financial, quality, and market targets is reviewed and action initiatives created when necessary.

- Revenue and direct expense levels are reviewed for each service line to identify opportunities for improvement, with specific targets for improvement established.
- Market data for each service line are reviewed by zip code to determine optimal growth locations for both volume and margin.
- Physician partners are supportive of and engaged in the service line review process for their programs. Their advice and support are sought out and integrated into program planning.
- Service lines identified as growth opportunities are assigned short- and long-term strategies, which are developed in concert with the physicians involved in providing those services.
- Physician partners are engaged in a cost reduction initiative as partners in improvement.
- Service lines and services are discontinued or scaled back either for lack of fit with the organization's mission or vision or because they continuously fail to achieve performance expectations.
- Resources are allocated on the basis of current and expected future performance of the service line, including investment in those services to build volume.
- In concert with physician partners, quality scores for each service line are monitored on an ongoing basis, with a goal of developing competitive advantage.
- Customer satisfaction scores are reviewed on a regular basis with the active engagement of all stakeholders in creating competitive advantage.

The three levers presented in this chapter pertain to strategic changes to a health system's service portfolio. They include the following:

- *Service outsourcing*—contracting with an external provider to offer an existing service on the organization's behalf
- *Service divestment*—discontinuing the provision of a program or service
- *Continuum realignment*—expanding the portfolio to include new services along the continuum of care or investing additional resources in an existing service

Portfolio-related decisions such as these are strategically important and often disruptive to the organization. For these reasons, leaders need a disciplined, unbiased review process to ensure that the organization consistently makes the right portfolio decisions for the future.

PORTFOLIO REVIEW

Healthcare leaders often spend considerable time planning and justifying the need for new programs and services. Once these programs are launched, many executive teams fail to retrospectively review performance and outcomes, or check to see if the initial assumptions about the program were correct or remain valid.

Portfolio review is a continuous, structured process by which organizations evaluate the performance of programs, departments, and services. Rather than looking solely for incremental improvement opportunities, portfolio review answers fundamental questions about how services are performed and determines how or whether these services should be considered for inclusion in the future portfolio.

Portfolio management ensures the following:

- Each program or service is aligned with its primary role in supporting the organization's success model.

- Capital and other resources are allocated across the enterprise in a manner that minimizes both over- and underinvestment.
- Programs continue to meet external market needs or support critical services in the organization.
- The organization makes objective, well-informed decisions when evaluating and implementing new programs and services.

Portfolio review is often conducted as a precursor to large performance improvement (PI) initiatives. A detailed assessment of each service area can set the stage for identifying services to grow toward improving cost and margin performance.

Portfolio decisions should be informed by current information on program performance, cost, and revenues. Service portfolio review should begin by compiling up-to-date performance information for each clinical service. Portfolio analysis data should include the following:

- Operating expenses and staffing levels, to size the current level of investment
- Profit and loss information, to understand margin performance
- Performance to budget, to understand how planned performance compares to actual performance
- Benchmarking data, to identify improvement opportunities
- Satisfaction data, to gauge how well customers' needs are met
- Market data, to understand the potential for growth in the service

Portfolio review should maintain consistency in how data are collected and reported across programs. Exhibit 10.1 illustrates the kind of baseline analysis that should be undertaken and the data summarized for any clinical program under review.

Performance expectations depend, in part, on the service and its function in the organization. Each component of the clinical service portfolio plays a role in supporting the organization's larger

Exhibit 10.1: Baseline Portfolio Review Components

Performance Dimension	Category	Questions
Revenue and growth	Revenues	• What are the projected net revenues for the current fiscal year? How do these projections compare with budgeted revenues for the same period? • What were the total net revenues for the previous 3 years, and how do they compare with this year's projected total? • How much downstream revenue is generated by this program?
	Patient volumes	• What are the projected patient volumes (e.g., cases, visits) for the current fiscal year? • How do these projected volumes compare with budgeted volumes for the same period? • What were the total volumes for the previous 3 years, and how do they compare with this year's projected total?
	Revenue per UOS	• What is the current vs. budgeted revenue per UOS? • How does the current revenue per UOS compare with previous years?
Operating expenses	Labor	• What are the FYTD total paid FTEs for the program? • How do FYTD FTEs compare with budgeted staffing? • What are the FYTD productive hours per UOS, and how does this trend compare with previous years? • How does current hours per UOS compare with external performance benchmarks? • What are the projected labor expenses for the current year, and how do they compare with the budget?
	Total expenses	• What are the projected total expenses for the current fiscal year? How do these projections compare with budgeted expenses for the same period? • What is the current vs. budgeted expense per UOS? • How does this expense compare with the previous 3 years? • How does current expense per UOS compare with external performance benchmarks?

(continued)

(continued from previous page)

Exhibit 10.1: Baseline Portfolio Review Components

Performance Dimension	Category	Questions
Profit and loss	Profitability	• What is the projected contribution margin of this program for the current fiscal year? • How does this margin compare with previous years, in total and on a per UOS basis? • What is the projected operating margin of this program for the current fiscal year (factoring in indirect allocated costs)? • How does this margin compare with previous years, in total and on a per UOS basis?
Market performance	Market share	• What is the program's current market share in the organization's core market? • What are the market awareness and perceptions of the program in contrast to competitors?
	Market growth	• What are the 5-year market growth projections for this program in the organization's core market?
	Consumer satisfaction	• How do consumers currently rate the program by overall satisfaction? • How do current satisfaction levels compare with previous years? • How likely are consumers to recommend the program to others?
Clinical quality performance	Quality	• How well is the program performing in terms of key clinical quality metrics? • How does current quality performance compare with the previous 3 years?

Note: FTE = full-time equivalent; FYTD = fiscal year to date; UOS = unit of service.

business success model. All clinical services and programs should support one or more components of that emerging success model by

- enhancing the organization's brand,
- building patient volumes and revenues, or
- generating sufficient operating margins.

Enhance the Organization's Brand

Some programs and services operate primarily to enhance the organization's brand in the community or support the corporate mission. These services typically have low contribution margins (revenue exceeding direct variable costs) and rarely have positive operating margins (revenue exceeding total allocated costs). Frequently, these services are a component of a health system's service line, for example:

- Ambulatory care clinics for low-income patients
- Graduate medical education and teaching programs
- Patient and community education programs
- Community health screenings
- Wellness programs
- Clinical research
- Hospice care

Build Patient Volumes and Revenues

Many of a health system's clinical programs serve a primary role of attracting and serving additional patients. In most cases, these services are revenue-producing programs that generate contribution margin but little or no operating margin. They are necessary for attracting new patients and steer referrals to downstream providers. Most acute care is included in this category, as inpatient cases usually contribute to overhead but do not generate operating income.

Volume-focused departments

- are essential sources of patient referrals to the organization's emergency services, primary care practices, urgent care centers, and so on;

- generate contribution margin, as with most acute care services, labor and delivery, home health services, wound care, dialysis, and others; and
- provide clinical and ancillary support to inpatient care, such as in pharmacy, laboratory, medical imaging, respiratory therapy, and rehabilitative therapy.

Generate Operating Margin

All organizations require sufficient operating margin to fund reinvestment and growth. For healthcare systems, operating margin is achieved by building high-revenue patient care service lines, managing the revenue cycle, and controlling expenses. Margin-producing functions typically include the following:

- Inpatient and outpatient surgery and endoscopy procedures
- Outpatient testing, such as imaging, laboratory, cardiac services, and neurological diagnostics
- Outpatient rehabilitation
- Inpatient service lines (with a focus on high-margin services)
- Specialty physician practices

Acute care services usually offer a combination of brand, volume, and margin contributions. Inpatient portfolio analysis should include case stratification and analysis by service line. Exhibit 10.2 is an example of a contribution margin analysis for inpatient spine cases. Using case-level cost accounting, this organization measures direct costs and contribution margin by diagnosis-related group to understand which type of cases provide operating margin and which build patient volume and contribute to margin.

A similar profit-and-loss analysis should be conducted for outpatient services and other components of the portfolio. Using this

Exhibit 10.2: Example of an Inpatient Service Line Contribution Analysis

Service Line	No. of Cases	Net Revenues	Direct Cost	CM ($)	CM (%)	Indirect Cost	OM ($)	OM (%)
Orthopedics	2,460	$55,657,974	$21,416,967	$34,241,007	62%	$17,218,825	$17,022,182	31%
Spine	954	$37,271,748	$13,513,986	$23,757,762	64%	$12,456,875	$11,300,887	30%
Thoracic surgery	213	$5,244,492	$2,304,461	$2,940,031	56%	$2,024,043	$915,988	17%
Neurosurgery	120	$3,515,764	$1,632,987	$1,882,777	54%	$1,319,465	$563,312	16%
Neurology	1,020	$10,007,211	$4,682,206	$5,325,005	53%	$4,174,049	$1,150,956	12%
Transplant	193	$29,161,831	$16,760,583	$12,401,248	43%	$9,858,955	$2,542,293	9%
Ophthalmology	27	$204,467	$97,826	$106,641	52%	$91,965	$14,676	7%
Other trauma	88	$635,940	$314,293	$321,647	51%	$283,978	$37,669	6%
Cardiac services	4,745	$117,615,375	$61,489,213	$56,126,162	48%	$50,585,288	$5,540,874	5%
General surgery	1,877	$66,119,963	$34,689,040	$31,430,923	48%	$28,710,714	$2,720,209	4%
General medicine	7,194	$71,035,675	$37,537,212	$33,498,463	47%	$33,642,493	–$144,030	0%
Urology	285	$4,236,826	$2,396,181	$1,840,645	43%	$1,892,341	–$51,696	–1%
Oncology	2,260	$35,691,625	$20,158,120	$15,533,505	44%	$16,563,043	–$1,029,538	–3%
Neonatology	2,609	$20,077,804	$12,567,568	$7,510,236	37%	$9,568,753	–$2,058,517	–10%
Vascular services	799	$17,698,915	$12,540,000	$5,158,915	29%	$7,830,227	–$2,671,312	–15%
ENT	156	$1,128,748	$708,881	$419,867	37%	$672,321	–$252,454	–22%
Gynecology	219	$1,710,508	$956,875	$753,633	44%	$1,047,315	–$293,682	–17%
Obstetrics	2,601	$16,543,867	$12,536,786	$4,007,081	24%	$11,700,409	–$7,693,328	–47%
Total	**27,820**	**$493,558,733**	**$256,303,185**	**$237,255,548**	**48%**	**$209,641,059**	**$27,614,489**	**6%**

Note: CM = contribution margin; ENT = ears, nose, and throat; OM = operating margin.

information, an executive team can evaluate each service and identify programs that

- warrant additional investment, as for programs that represent revenue growth opportunities or areas that are undercapitalized;
- need cost improvement to occur to build margin or achieve benchmark performance;
- should retain current investment levels, referring to departments and programs that are operating at acceptable performance levels and should remain unaltered;
- should be delivered in a different manner, as through outsourcing to another organization, joint venturing with another entity, or altering processes to provide programs in a different way; and
- should be divested, as when internal or external factors have rendered the service unnecessary or difficult to sustain.

PORTFOLIO COLLABORATIVE TEAMS

Large PI initiatives frequently include collaborative teams focused on portfolio management opportunities. The strategic nature of portfolio review necessitates that the team include senior leaders. Portfolio teams must conduct, or have access to, significant program-level financial analysis; market assessments; and other decision support information.

Portfolio collaborative teams are responsible for the following:

- Inventorying the organization's service portfolio and narrowing the focus to a subset of programs with the highest potential for improvement
- Gathering current and historical data on financial and market performance

- Collecting additional information from department leaders, physicians, and other stakeholders on program issues and opportunities
- Evaluating interventions and selecting those that will most accelerate a program's performance

Portfolio teams should follow a structured review process (exhibit 10.3), beginning with an assessment of the program's financial performance. Determining the best options for a program depends on its functional role. On the basis of this principle, the team should identify cost improvement opportunities that are required to build margin and profitability. In some cases, this increase can only occur through outsourcing to or partnering with external providers. In other cases, a program should be divested.

In addition to cost improvement, the portfolio team should identify opportunities for growing market share for programs that enhance patient volume and operating margin. These opportunities may require the organization to make additional capacity investments to accommodate growth.

Exhibit 10.4 is a guide for leading teams through the portfolio decision process. By addressing specific questions on comparative cost performance, profitability, and market opportunities, a team can gauge a program's current performance relative to that program's required role in the business success model.

NONCLINICAL PORTFOLIO REVIEW

Portolio management principles can apply as well to nonclinical services and departments. A health system's administrative and support functions help it achieve favorable outcomes in patient care and service quality. These functions shape and enhance the organization's brand and community reputation, both of which steer patients, payers, physicians, and workers to the health system.

Exhibit 10.3: Portfolio Review Decision Process

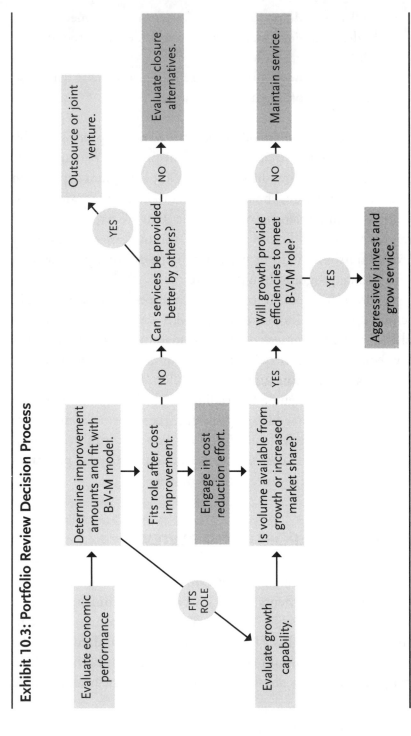

Note: B-V-M = brand, volume, and margin.

Specifically, these programs

- enhance the brand and image of the organization through public and governmental relations, marketing, and the organization's philanthropic foundation;
- provide leadership direction and set the organization's culture via administrative services, human resources, mission services, and other administrative areas;
- maintain a safe, patient-centered care environment, as with environmental services, maintenance, security, infection control, biomedical engineering, and sterile processing;
- improve clinical and service outcomes through the medical staff office, training and development, PI, and risk management;
- maintain valid data and information to support patient care via medical records, information services, patient registration, clinical documentation improvement, and others;
- provide customer services to patients and families via telecommunications, the cafeteria, the gift shop, patient relations, and valet and parking services;
- manage patient access, throughput, and placement via patient scheduling, case management, social services, patient registration, and the physician referral call center;
- manage the organization's operating expenses and utilization through functions such as accounting and budgeting, PI, utilization review, case management, and materials management; and
- sustain the organization's revenue and cash flow via the business office, collections, and patient registration.

Portfolio teams may evaluate a combination of clinical and non-clinical programs as part of their charter. In the process, these teams frequently identify services that have cost or margin improvement

Exhibit 10.4: Clinical Portfolio Evaluation Matrix

Improvement Strategy	Primary Service Role		
	Enhances Organizational Brand	Builds Contribution Margin and Patient Volume	Sustains Operating Margin
Invest or grow	• Additional investment is needed to improve brand position in the community. • Investment is required to close significant quality or safety gaps. • Investment is required to sustain the organization's teaching/research mission. • Investment is required to meet an unmet need in the community.	• Additional investment will result in increased referrals to high-margin programs. • Opportunities are available to grow share in the organization's core market. • The service is critical to supporting population health initiatives. • Investment is required to improve clinical and service quality.	• Additional investment will result in higher operating margins for the organization. • Opportunities are available to grow the service in the organization's core market. • The service is critical to supporting population health initiatives. • Investment is required to improve clinical and service quality.
Improve contribution margin	• Additional external funding is available to offset expenses. • Opportunities are available to lower operating expenses for this program.	• Benchmark data show opportunities for cost improvement for this program. • The program has excess capacity and can accommodate increased patient volumes. • The program has negative or lower-than-expected contribution margin.	• Opportunity is available to improve operating and contribution margins through cost improvements. • Benchmark data show opportunities for cost improvement. • The program has lower-than-expected operating margin and needs to improve.

(continued)

(continued from previous page)

Exhibit 10.4: Clinical Portfolio Evaluation Matrix

Improvement Strategy	Primary Service Role		
	Enhances Organizational Brand	Builds Contribution Margin and Patient Volume	Sustains Operating Margin
Maintain	• The program has effectively enhanced the organization's brand and mission without overinvestment.	• The program provides sufficient referrals to other programs; additional investment will not result in more referrals. • The program compares favorably to cost benchmarks; opportunity for improvement in contribution margin is limited.	• Benchmark data show limited opportunities for cost improvement. • The program already has high operating margins.
Outsource or joint venture	• The program can be delivered more effectively (lower cost, higher market effectiveness, higher quality, etc.) through outsourcing or partnership with an outside entity.	• The program can be delivered more effectively (lower cost, higher revenues, higher quality, etc.) through a sourcing agreement with an outside organization.	• The program can be delivered more effectively (lower cost, higher revenues, higher quality, etc.) through a sourcing agreement with an outside organization.
Divest	• The program has failed to build the organization's brand or sustain the mission. • External funding is no longer available to support this program.	• The program has failed to provide enough downstream business or contribution margin to warrant continuation. • External demand or funding for this program has dropped or been eliminated.	• Scale of business is insufficient to enable the program to achieve a minimum contribution margin threshold.

opportunities in productivity, supply, or utilization that can be pursued by other teams or initiatives.

For some programs, a portfolio team may determine that the best approach for improvement is to offer the service in a different manner or to exit the service entirely. This type of adjustment involves the use of the remaining three improvement levers discussed in this book:

- Service outsourcing
- Service divestment
- Continuum realignment

LEVER 16: SERVICE OUTSOURCING

Organizations often perform services and functions that are necessary to their business, but they may not have the resources or experience to deliver the services in an optimal manner. Financial conditions or events, such as the loss of a leader, the need for significant capital infusion, or continuously low performance, may require executive leadership to consider other options for service delivery.

Outsourcing represents the "make versus buy" improvement option of portfolio management. Many organizations elect to source programs and functions to external companies with the expertise and focus to provide the service effectively. Outsourcing is a common strategy employed by organizations to reduce operating expenses, particularly in noncore, support, and administrative services.

Sourcing firms usually have the scale, expertise, and labor resources to provide a service at lower costs than can be achieved by the health system. As illustrated in exhibit 10.5, sourcing organizations use their expertise and focus to produce high levels of productivity and lowered payroll expenses. Their scale of operation can also enable lower costs for supplies and other purchasing expenses.

Exhibit 10.5: Sources of Cost Improvement Through Outsourcing

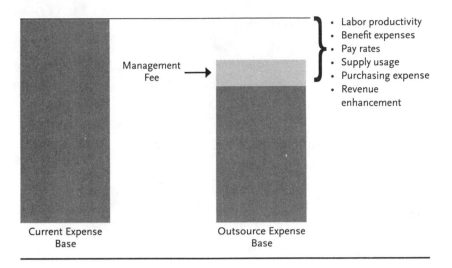

Cost savings is not the only driver of outsourcing decisions. Organizations also outsource services to firms to

- improve organizational focus on core services,
- gain access to best practices and technologies,
- obtain expertise and management talent that are difficult to attract and retain,
- free up internal resources and capital for redeployment to other priorities,
- share financial risk, and
- provide investment and cash infusion.

Outsourcing is ubiquitous in the healthcare industry. Many health systems contract with outside organizations to provide support and select administrative services. Outsourcing can occur at the department level (e.g., the public relations director hires a freelance writer to produce website copy) or on a larger scale (e.g., the hospital outsources most of the support service areas). The most frequently outsourced services include the following:

- Environmental services
- Dietary services
- Safety and security functions
- Engineering and maintenance functions
- Construction
- Grounds keeping
- Release of information (medical records)
- Transcription services
- Patient accounts and collections functions
- Biomedical engineering services
- Laundry and linen services
- Materials management
- Reference laboratory services
- Public relations

Outsourcing decisions should be supported by an economic evaluation of the current state versus the proposed outsourced state. This analysis should account for current direct operating costs as well as expected future costs such as needed capital and technology investments or facility upgrades. The ability to lower opportunity costs, such as by freeing up staffing and space for other purposes, should also factor into the analysis.

Outsourcing decisions frequently result in the displacement of internal staff who currently perform the work. An important consideration is to gain an understanding of and to plan for the cultural and morale impact and potential separation costs that can occur when a service is sourced to an outside organization.

Outsourcing does not remedy all of an organization's operational issues and challenges, but it can be the right choice for some components of the service portfolio. The key aspects of outsourcing for leaders to understand are the operational benefits that support outsourcing, the ability to find the sourcing partner that that fits culturally with the organization, and the navigation of staff and customers through the transition.

Likewise, portfolio review should evaluate programs and services that are currently outsourced. Changing business conditions can create opportunities to bring outsourced services back inside the organization. The evaluation of insourcing should follow a similar process to analyze costs and service demand and to identify issues and expenses associated with the transition.

Joint Ventures and Partnerships

As an alternative to outsourcing, many healthcare systems develop joint ventures and other partnerships with other provider organizations. Joint ventures are common in clinical service provision and have a primary benefit of spreading financial risk with other entities. Clinical program joint ventures are established with regularity between health systems and physician groups. Such agreements are useful tools for aligning hospitals and affiliated physicians, particularly in ambulatory clinical services. Health systems may also partner with other hospital groups, including competitors, to provide joint programs and services to local communities.

LEVER 17: SERVICE DIVESTMENT

For some programs, services, or entities, the best improvement option may be to shut down the service or sell it to another organization. Health systems usually divest patient care services, community programs, grant-funded initiatives, or facilities that no longer fit effectively in the organization's portfolio. Frequently, these decisions are precipitated by changing market conditions or economic issues, as with the following examples:

- An outreach program has lost the funding that had sustained it in the past.
- A joint venture with a physician's group has been dissolved.
- An outpatient surgery facility has struggled for years to break even in a highly competitive market.
- A hospital decides to close a child care center due to underutilization.
- A multihospital system decides to sell one of its hospitals to invest in a different market.
- A program that is struggling to build patient volumes is experiencing declining revenues and limited opportunities for incremental productivity improvement.

Service divestment decisions are rarely easy to implement. Eliminating programs and services can negatively affect patients and staff. Healthcare leaders must anticipate the impact of these decisions on constituent groups, communicate the decisions and the reasons for the change, and offer alternatives. Expected cost savings must be balanced with implementation costs, such as severance pay, lost revenues, and legal expense.

LEVER 18: CONTINUUM REALIGNMENT

Population health, accountable care, and risk-based payment are intended to improve clinical outcomes and costs by requiring providers to coordinate services across the care continuum. Consequently, the drive for enhanced care alignment has precipitated much of the structural alignment of providers. These changes are accelerating hospital consolidation and the formation of large regional health systems. Increasingly, health systems are expanding vertically to include physician services, post-acute care, and other components of the medical care continuum.

Healthcare systems look much different from the hospital-centric organizations of the past. Exhibit 10.6 contrasts the revenue profile of a traditional freestanding hospital with today's integrated healthcare system.

In the recent past, the acute care hospital, encircled by independent physician offices, was the model of most healthcare delivery. The traditional model has been altered by multiple factors and trends, including the following:

- A shift from acute care to ambulatory care
- Growth in rehabilitation and post-acute services
- Growth in home-based care
- A shift in nonemergent cases from hospital emergency departments to freestanding providers
- Acceleration in outpatient procedures performed in physician offices

Healthcare organizations have increasingly large and diverse service portfolios. The expanded service offerings include nontraditional programs requiring new leadership knowledge and skills. These services should be managed with the same portfolio management disciplines used with current programs.

Continuum realignment represents the myriad strategies employed by health systems to transition operations from a predominantly acute care model to an integrated care system that can deliver medical services along the full continuum of care. When effectively executed, a seamless care continuum can

- close care gaps for patients,
- improve the transition of patients across care sites and services,
- reduce the rate of readmissions and other off-quality outcomes, and
- add sources of revenue.

Exhibit 10.6: Traditional Hospital Revenue Profile Versus Integrated System Revenue Profile

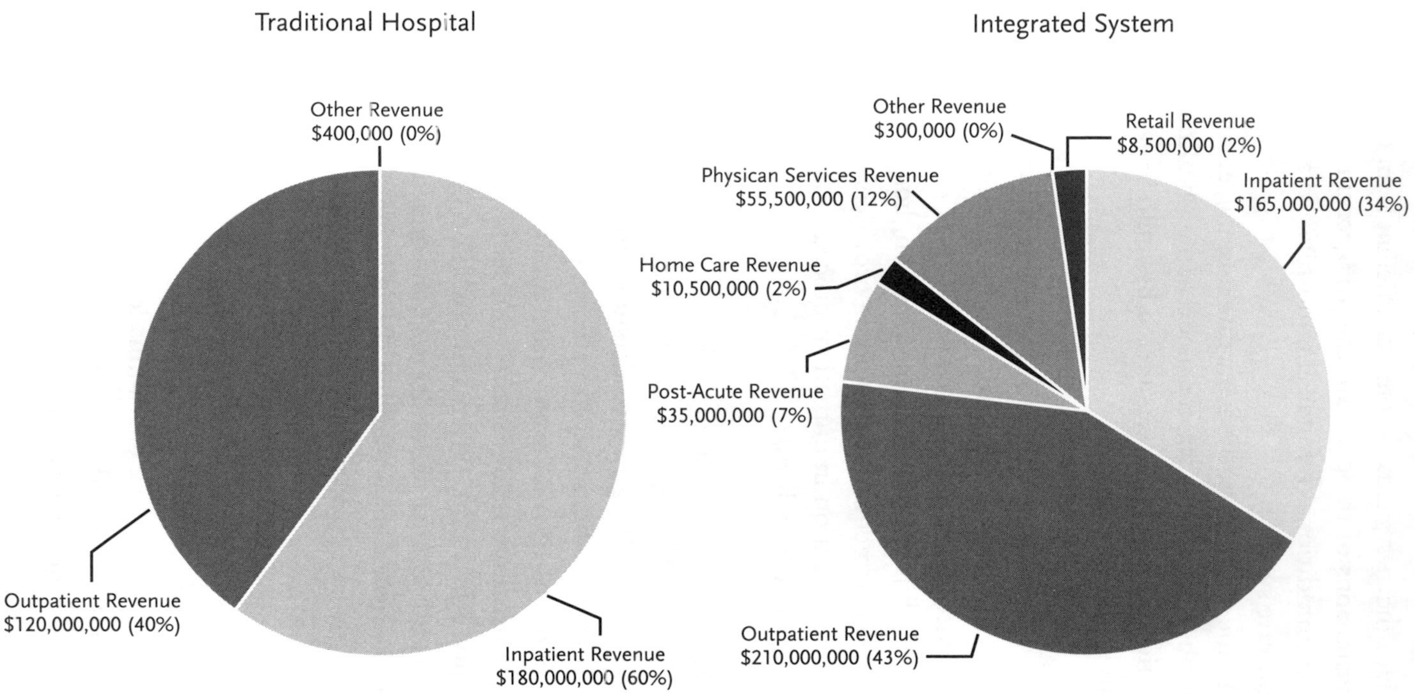

Integrated System

Inpatient Revenue
$165,000,000 (34%)

Retail Revenue
$8,500,000 (2%)

Other Revenue
$300,000 (0%)

Physican Services Revenue
$55,500,000 (12%)

Home Care Revenue
$10,500,000 (2%)

Post-Acute Revenue
$35,000,000 (7%)

Outpatient Revenue
$210,000,000 (43%)

Traditional Hospital

Inpatient Revenue
$180,000,000 (60%)

Other Revenue
$400,000 (0%)

Outpatient Revenue
$120,000,000 (40%)

An expanded service offering alters the dynamics of the portfolio management process. Continuum realignment brings new criteria and complexity to portfolio evaluation. When assessing a program, executives must account for the future value of the program in the emerging service portfolio. A profitable inpatient orthopedic service line, for example, will operate differently in the future as more surgeries shift to ambulatory settings. These shifts in care setting change how health systems are reimbursed and, consequently, alter the structure of and required investment in delivery systems. Factors such as these can significantly influence service line investments and cost-related decisions.

Consolidation has enabled large health systems to amass numerous physician practices, ambulatory programs, and post-acute services. Some organizations pursue provider-sponsored health plans with full-risk capabilities. Over time, these service portfolios typically shift, with some components growing and others retracting. Leaders need to review each component of the expanded service portfolio (exhibit 10.7) and determine the best alternative for providing the service.

Effective portfolio management requires leadership skills and expertise in attracting and aligning with high-value partners. According to Porter and Teisberg (2006), value in healthcare is created by doing a few things well. In operational terms, fulfillment of this mandate effectively awards portions of the care continuum to providers with the scale, experience, and focused expertise to produce the best quality outcomes at the lowest costs. Increasingly, health systems will serve as a "general contractor," determining which continuum services to "make" and which to "buy." These decisions will rest largely on the organization's scale and internal capabilities and on the availability of alternative, high-value providers in the local market.

Stand-alone hospitals and small health systems may not have the scale and resources to control the full care continuum. Many of these organizations will need to reduce their service portfolio and migrate

Exhibit 10.7: The Expanded Health System Service Portfolio

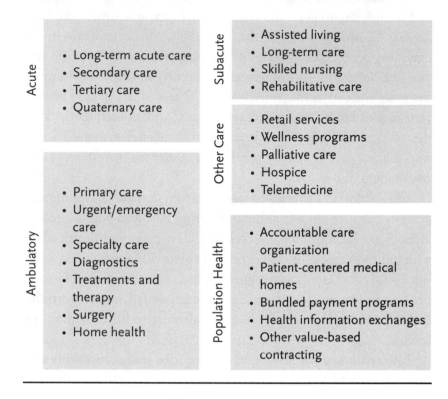

Acute
- Long-term acute care
- Secondary care
- Tertiary care
- Quaternary care

Ambulatory
- Primary care
- Urgent/emergency care
- Specialty care
- Diagnostics
- Treatments and therapy
- Surgery
- Home health

Subacute
- Assisted living
- Long-term care
- Skilled nursing
- Rehabilitative care

Other Care
- Retail services
- Wellness programs
- Palliative care
- Hospice
- Telemedicine

Population Health
- Accountable care organization
- Patient-centered medical homes
- Bundled payment programs
- Health information exchanges
- Other value-based contracting

to a focused factory (Herzlinger 1997) strategy. Providers that direct their energies on a narrow plane and execute well will be able to deliver differentiated clinical outcomes at significantly lower costs than those that insist on maintaining a broad portfolio. The approach is not without risks, however. A focused factory strategy requires the organization to dramatically reduce fixed costs and eliminate services. The organization must continually maintain differentiated quality for its primary services to outperform competing programs.

PART III

Design, Implementation, and Performance Monitoring

CHAPTER 11

Structure and Process for Performance Improvement

LARGE PERFORMANCE IMPROVEMENT (PI) initiatives require a project structure that defines individual roles and accountabilities and facilitates executive oversight and decision making. This structure is necessary to set priorities and targets, oversee the work of collaborative teams during redesign, and manage implementation.

As a final step of the assessment phase, the organization's executive team should form a steering committee. The steering committee should include those senior-level executives with broad responsibility and decision-making authority for operational and strategic performance. Frequently, the organization's senior leadership team serves as the steering committee, and the committee may also include individuals from human resources, PI, and similar support areas.

A steering committee has responsibility for the following:

- Identifying opportunities and setting cost, revenue, and other operational improvement targets
- Establishing collaborative teams and approving team charters
- Assigning team leaders and approving team membership
- Allocating internal and external resources to support initiatives

- Reviewing and approving collaborative team recommendations
- Affirming opportunity-sizing and risk-rating assessments at the conclusion of the redesign phase
- Approving implementation plans and driving implementation
- Overseeing communication with the board, the medical staff, and the rest of the organization about the PI

The steering committee is typically chaired by the CEO, the chief operating officer, or another member of the executive team.

Exhibit 11.1 is an example of how one healthcare system structured its organization-wide PI initiative. This organization launched six collaborative teams, each focused on a different improvement category. In several cases, team leaders assigned subteams focused on specific functional areas or business units. The productivity collaborative team, for example, included a human resources subteam focused on pay and benefit issues and labor policies. Additional subteams were assigned to pursue productivity performance opportunities in key operational areas, including nursing and surgery.

PERFORMANCE IMPROVEMENT COLLABORATIVE TEAMS

Improvement initiatives work best when led by multidisciplinary collaborative teams with defined charters and clear expectations. As a final step in the predesign phase, the steering committee should formulate and approve team charters for each identified initiative. The charter should delineate the primary objectives of the team, define the scope of the work, and identify performance goals and the expected timing of the impact.

Exhibit 11.2 provides an example of a team charter format for a collaborative team focused on service regionalization opportunities. Usually, a collaborative team is assigned an economic goal (cost

Exhibit 11.1: Example of a Performance Improvement Initiative Structure

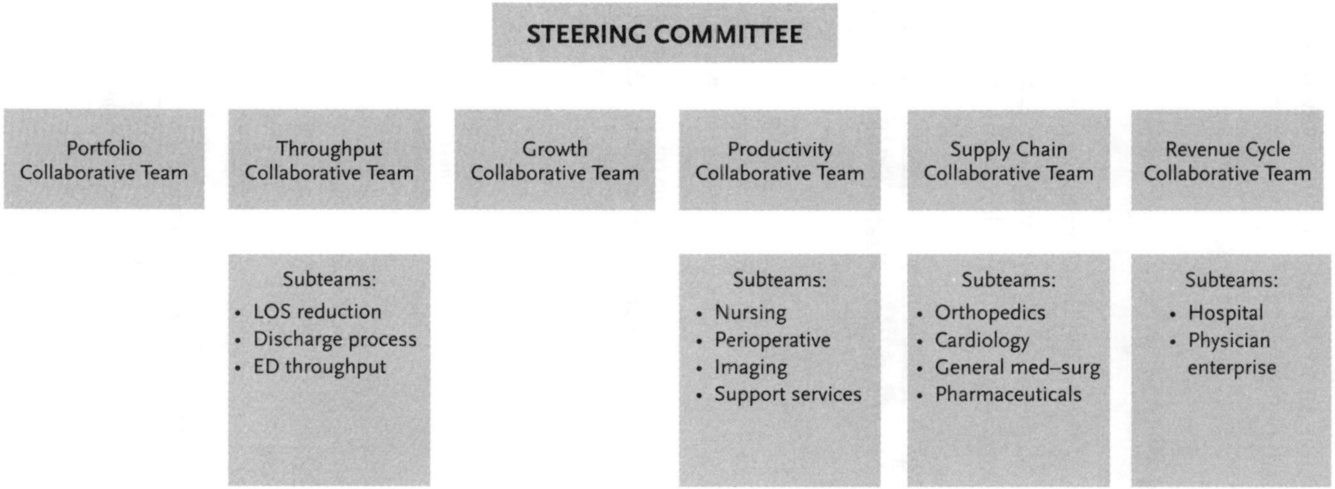

STEERING COMMITTEE

| Portfolio Collaborative Team | Throughput Collaborative Team | Growth Collaborative Team | Productivity Collaborative Team | Supply Chain Collaborative Team | Revenue Cycle Collaborative Team |

Throughput Collaborative Team — Subteams:
- LOS reduction
- Discharge process
- ED throughput

Productivity Collaborative Team — Subteams:
- Nursing
- Perioperative
- Imaging
- Support services

Supply Chain Collaborative Team — Subteams:
- Orthopedics
- Cardiology
- General med–surg
- Pharmaceuticals

Revenue Cycle Collaborative Team — Subteams:
- Hospital
- Physician enterprise

Note: ED = emergency department; LOS = length of stay.

improvement, revenue growth, or both) to attain. Economic targets are often represented as annual amounts and may be defined as a range rather than a single figure.

THE REDESIGN PHASE

Successful performance redesign requires the active engagement of individuals who understand the processes and issues under review and have ultimate responsibility for implementing future changes.

Exhibit 11.2: Example of a Regionalization Collaborative Team Charter

Team objectives		• Review inventory listing of administrative and support programs and services across the region; validate current investment (labor and nonlabor) for each site.
		• Confirm decision criteria for evaluating service options; apply criteria to each service and program, and identify 10–15 programs with the highest potential for service improvement and cost savings.
		• Identify opportunities to leverage corporate services as a component of service delivery. Determine economic and service impact associated with these changes.
		• Identify risks and implementation issues associated with each recommended change.
		• Determine implementation sequence and glide path for years 1–3.
Current regional investment (estimated)	$200 million	• Based on last year's actual expenditures (labor and nonlabor) for an initial list of 30+ administrative and support service categories.
Economic target	$6 million–$10 million	• Based on an estimated 3–5% reduction in leadership payroll expense.
Timing of impact	Primarily years 2 and 3	• In many cases, program changes will need to be preceded by the establishment of regional leadership roles.
Other performance expectations		• Improve consistency of services across the system.

The steering committee identifies the individuals to lead and participate in the collaborative teams and approves the team membership.

Collaborative Team Roles

Collaborative teams are assigned standard roles with specific responsibilities (exhibit 11.3).

Executive Sponsor

A steering committee member should be assigned as an executive
sponsor for each collaborative team. The executive sponsor typically
has formal responsibility for the areas included in the team charter
and undertakes the following duties:

- Facilitate communication between the steering committee
  and the collaborative team.
- Periodically attend meetings and provide senior-level
  advice to the team.
- Remove obstacles over the course of the team's work.
- Challenge assumptions and biases of the team to produce
  optimal results.

Team Leader

Each collaborative team requires a designated leader to oversee and
facilitate the work of the group. Typically, the leader has operational
responsibilities in or content knowledge of the area under study.
Team leads may also be generalists with process knowledge and
facilitation expertise.

Team leaders undertake the following responsibilities:

- Identify and finalize team membership with guidance from
  the executive sponsor.
- Prepare and execute team agendas.
- Facilitate team meetings throughout the redesign process.

Exhibit 11.3: Standard Roles for Collaborative Teams

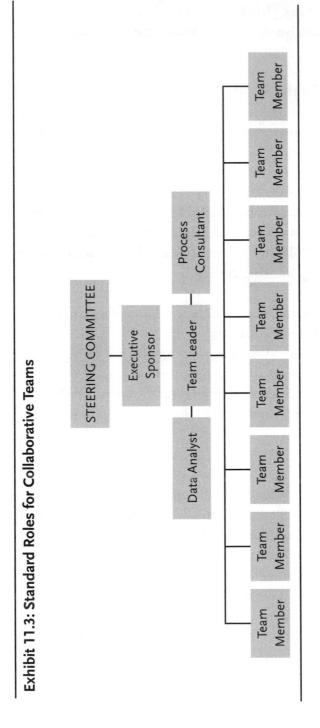

- Assign tasks and homework to team members.
- Work closely with the executive sponsor, and provide periodic progress reports.
- Oversee implementation plan development.
- Lead the development and presentation of findings and redesign recommendations to the steering committee.

Team Members

Team members are selected on the basis of their formal roles, content knowledge, creativity and analytical skills, and ability to work productively with others. Team members should include representatives from all major functional areas under review.

Team members are expected to contribute in the following ways:

- Actively participate in all meetings.
- Help diagnose process issues and identify causal factors.
- Complete assignments between meetings.
- Identify and develop potential redesign solutions.
- Facilitate communication with individuals and areas external to the team.
- Assist with implementation as directed.

Team members may be assigned to head subteams focused on specific areas or process issues. Subteam leads have responsibility for completing their assigned tasks and reporting back to the core team.

Team Support

A collaborative team should be supported by a data analyst with proficiencies in benchmarking, financial analysis, and decision support. The analyst is responsible for collecting and interpreting data, sizing economic opportunities identified by the collaborative team, and validating the calculations and risk ratings of each recommendation.

When available, a process consultant should be assigned to support collaborative teams. A process consultant

- helps facilitate meetings and supports the team leader,
- provides consulting support and team training regarding improvement tools and techniques,
- provides expertise in change management and organizational communication, and
- delivers management support for implementation planning and execution.

THE COLLABORATIVE TEAM PROCESS

A collaborative team is responsible for achieving the objectives delineated by the team charter. During the redesign phase, the collaborative team undertakes the following activities:

- Evaluate current processes and systems to reveal where performance is lacking.
- Collect relevant performance data to support findings and recommendations.
- Brainstorm ideas, interventions, and solutions for addressing performance issues.
- Vet ideas and determine the subset of solutions that are the best alternatives for the organization.
- Size and risk-rate each recommended opportunity.
- Prepare a draft implementation plan.
- Present findings and recommendations to the steering committee.

A collaborative team typically meets over a six- to eight-week period with sessions scheduled for ninety minutes to two hours. To keep the process on track, collaborative teams should have the following characteristics:

- *Accountable*, with clearly defined roles and responsibilities for each team participant

- *Structured*, with an improvement process and team approach that is understood by everyone involved
- *Data driven*, whereby conclusions and decisions are based on information and fact rather than perceptions and anecdotal information
- *Focused*, with an emphasis on identifying core issues and solutions in the scope of the team charter rather than functioning as an open-ended forum for debate or to rehash problems without definitive solutions
- *Time limited*, with defined target dates for completion

Exhibit 11.4 depicts a six-meeting process for a productivity collaborative team supported by several functional subteams. This example specifies what activities take place at each meeting and what actions are taken between meetings. Other types of collaborative teams follow similar processes, although the content of the meetings, the use of subteams, and other factors vary.

Meeting 1 serves to orient the team and equip the subteam leaders to lead their groups. Team members should leave this meeting with a clear understanding of why the initiative was formed and what goals were established for the team. During the meeting, which is often considered the kickoff event for the initiative, members are given an overview of the PI framework and the 18 improvement levers. Additional reference materials about the model are provided for team members to review outside the meetings.

To stay on an accelerated schedule, task assignments must be completed between meetings. The team leader assigns homework, with deadlines, to team members. This assignment may include additional data gathering, clarification on process issues, input from individuals who are not part of the team, or assignments for subteams. Most of the quantitative analysis to support team discussion is performed between meetings by the data analyst.

As a homework assignment after meeting 1, each productivity core team member is asked to compile a list of organizational issues and gaps that contribute to low productivity. Each team member should

Exhibit 11.4: Example of a Collaborative Productivity Team's Six-Meeting Process

Meeting 1	• Review initial benchmarking and productivity assessment results. • Review team targets and timeline. • Confirm charters, scope, and membership of subteams. • Train team members and subteam leaders on improvement model and 18 improvement levers. • Train team on methodology for opportunity sizing and risk rating. • Homework: Assess system and process gaps that impede productivity.
Between meetings	• Launch productivity subteams (meeting 1). • Complete homework assignments. • Review handout materials on the improvement model and levers.
Meeting 2	• Homework report-out: Identify organizational gaps that impede productivity performance. • Brainstorm improvement opportunities to close competency gaps. • Discuss themes, issues, and opportunities arising from subteam leaders' meeting 1 status report. • Identify quick wins and record them on tracking sheet. • Identify issues for communication to the organization.
Between meetings	• Initiate subteams' meeting 2. • Quantify opportunities identified by the team (analysts). • Communicate progress to the organization.
Meeting 3	• Finalize recommendations on competency gap closure; quantify opportunities. • Subteam report-out: Discuss initial opportunities that have been identified. • Identify quick wins. • Brainstorm organization-wide productivity improvement opportunities.
Between meetings	• Initiate subteams' meeting 3. • Provide the steering committee with an update on progress (executive sponsor).

(continued)

(continued from previous page)

Exhibit 11.4: Example of a Collaborative Productivity Team's Six-Meeting Process

Meeting 4	• Receive feedback from steering committee delivered by executive sponsor. • Receive updates and report-outs from each subteam. • Brainstorm organization-wide productivity improvement opportunities. • Review and validate calculated opportunity and risk rating on tracking sheet. • Provide feedback to subteams for moving forward. • Identify enablers that support recommendations.
Between meetings	• Initiate subteams' meeting 4. • Quantify opportunities identified by subteams. • Communicate progress to the organization.
Meeting 5	• Receive updates and report-outs from each subteam. • Review and validate calculated opportunity and risk rating. • Develop initial draft of consolidated tracking sheet; check calculated opportunity against team target. • Identify enablers that will support recommendations.
Between meetings	• Complete final quantification (subteams) and provide to subteam leader.
Meeting 6	• Finalize tracking sheet, and validate sizing and risk rating for each line item. • Formulate additional process, enabler, and system recommendations for improving productivity performance. • Discuss implementation planning, and assign responsibilities for completion. • Discuss presentation to steering committee.
After meeting 6	• Complete implementation plan. • Present recommendations to steering committee. • Finalize and implement plan.

complete the assignment and plan to discuss the lists at meeting 2. This exercise can yield important insights into systemic issues that must be addressed by the organization to improve performance.

Beginning in meeting 2, the core team focuses on policy and systemwide issues and opportunities that affect labor productivity performance across all departments and functions. These issues may include the following:

- Control of overtime
- Use of agency and contracted labor
- Pay policies, including
  - shift and weekend differentials,
  - on-call and call-back pay, and
  - holiday pay
- Benefit costs, including
  - health benefits,
  - life insurance, and
  - tuition reimbursement
- Adherence to labor budget standards and benchmark targets
- Staff turnover rates and associated costs
- Position control processes and systems

The team brainstorms ideas for improving organizational performance in each of these areas. For example, the team may identify opportunities to lower overtime usage from 3 percent to 2.5 percent of total paid hours by focusing on staff scheduling practices in departments that tend to exceed overtime usage benchmarks. Prior to meeting 2, leaders and facilitators should review brainstorming principles and techniques to fully leverage the power of the process, remembering that all ideas are welcomed and documented, everyone participates, and judging is reserved for the risk-rating phase. This process continues in meetings 3 through 5. The team evaluates each performance area, estimates the economic impact of each solution, and rates the difficulty of implementation.

The subteams' launches occur immediately after meeting 1. The subteams identify improvements for specific functional areas or departments. These opportunities support achievement of the core team's overall economic target. These groups meet four or five times using a similar meeting structure and methodology as the core team. As findings and recommendations emerge, subteams report out during meetings 3 through 6 of the core productivity collaborative team. The subteam leader typically provides the report but, if necessary, can be joined by other members of the subteam.

The subteams focus their redesign efforts on those PI levers that are most applicable to the functions under review. Appendix B is a listing of key functional areas and the subset of improvement levers that are most applicable for the function. This list is intended as a tool to help teams focus on opportunities with high economic yield and impact on service and quality. Other levers may provide incremental benefit as well and should be considered when opportunities arise.

Quick Wins

In the course of a team's work, some ideas emerge that

- carry low implementation risk,
- generate immediate savings,
- involve a limited scope of change,
- can enable other improvements to occur, or
- do not require the approval of the executive committee to implement.

These "quick win" opportunities should be vetted by the subteams and presented to the core team for inclusion on the tracking template and counted toward the team's improvement target.

Quick wins are beneficial because they create momentum for change and generate immediate improvement and cost savings for the organization. Additionally, quick wins provide motivational success early in the life of a team.

Tracking Templates

To be successful, collaborative teams require a consistent tool and methodology to record improvement ideas and to size opportunities. Exhibit 11.5 is an example of a tracking tool for a surgical services productivity collaborative team. This template is used to record all improvement ideas generated by the team. Over the course of several meetings, the team evaluates and rules out some ideas, eliminates or combines duplicates, and quantifies the opportunities for recommended improvement.

Each line item represents a discrete improvement idea corresponding to a specific improvement lever. Succinct descriptions of the proposed changes are necessary so that the steering committee and other external audiences understand the recommendation in precise terms. Additional clarification or assumptions can be recorded in the notes section.

For each item, the team calculates the expected economic impact of the opportunity by first ranking solutions by an estimated order or range of magnitude before calculating a precise measure. This approach helps the team focus on high-impact solutions and avoid spending significant time on quantifying small opportunities. This amount is usually reflected as annual savings and should represent savings net of any investment requirements or risk adjustment. The data analyst calculates the savings opportunity with input from the team members. The team should ensure that savings calculations are not duplicated in other line items and unearth hidden costs that may be transferred to another part of the organization.

Next, the calculated annual savings are adjusted by the team to account for potential risks associated with implementation. Risk adjustment should be neither too conservative nor too aggressive.

Highly conservative estimates can be perceived as timid and may reduce the perceived urgency for change. Conversely, aggressive estimates can be perceived as unrealistic and increase the risk of missing targets.

One method of risk assessment involves gauging the implementation preparedness of the organization by posing a few key questions. In exhibit 11.5, the team asks the following questions for each initiative:

- Does the organization have previous experience in effecting similar change in this area or function?
- Is completion of the improvement intervention within the control of the organization, or does it depend on the cooperation of patients, physicians, or external organizations?
- Does the organization presently have the skills and abilities to implement the proposed changes?

If the answer to all the questions is "Yes," the spreadsheet calculates 80 percent of the opportunity, recorded as the risk-rated annualized run rate impact. If one or two of the questions are answered "No," 50 percent of the opportunity is calculated. If all three are answered "No," only 20 percent of the opportunity is recorded.

Risk ratings are an important factor when presenting recommendations to the steering committee. Members of the committee must understand the rationale for high risk ratings; in some cases, senior leaders can help remove some of the risk factors prior to implementation, leading to changes in the risk rating (e.g., change reds to yellows and yellows to green, represented as varying shades of gray in exhibit 11.5) and increased projected economic gain.

As a final adjustment, the expected savings during the current budget year should be reflected as appropriate. Some initiatives take longer to implement than others, and understanding when savings are expected to accrue is important. In the template example (exhibit

Exhibit 11.5: Example of a Surgical Services Collaborative Team Tracking Sheet

Department	Item	Improvement Lever	Item Description	Units of Improvement	Value per Unit of Improvement	Annualized Run-Rate Impact	Is There a Prior History of Success in This Area?	Is Completion in Our Control?	Do Skills Currently Exist to Complete?
Main operating room	1	Management restructuring	1 supervisor position on day shift will be vacant as of 4/11. We will not fill this position.	1.0 FTE	$65,000	$65,000	Yes	Yes	Yes
PACU	2	Process improvement	Improve throughput in PACU; lower staff through 20% reduction in PACU LOS by 20%.	1.5 FTEs	$52,000/FTE	$78,000	Yes	Yes	Yes
Main operating room	3	Dynamic staffing	Reconfigure the afternoon staff schedule; reduce no. of teams on Tu. and Thu. to reflect drop-off in afternoon cases.	2.0 FTEs	$45,000/FTE	$90,000	Yes	Yes	Yes
Main operating room	4	Demand smoothing	Reconfigure block scheduling for orthopedic and spine cases to better balance cases across the week.	1.6 FTEs	$52,000/FTE	$83,200	Yes	No	Yes
ASU	5	Service divestment	Eliminate Saturday schedule in ASU.	4.0 FTEs	$43,000/FTE	$172,000	No	No	No
ASU/main operating room	6	Growth	New general surgeons are expected to bring in 20 added cases per week starting 5/1.	1,040 additional cases per year	$2,300 CM per case	$2,392,000	Yes	No	Yes
				Totals		$2,880,200			

(continued)

(continued from previous page)

Exhibit 11.5: Example of a Surgical Services Collaborative Team Tracking Sheet

Department	Risk Rating	Risk-Rated Annualized Run Rate Impact	Current FY Months	Risk-Rated Current FY Cash Impact	Assigned to	Notes
Main operating room	Green	$52,000	10	$43,333	Cindy	We will need to reassign workload among the remaining supervisors; may need to shift some supply chain responsibilities to clerical staff.
PACU	Green	$62,400	8	$41,600	Leigh Ann	May take 3–4 months before we achieve the target LOS.
Main operating room	Green	$72,000	8	$48,000	Paula	Have to work through scheduling preferences with some staff.
Main operating room	Yellow	$41,600	9	$31,200	Cindy	Need to get buy-in from the ortho surgeons; could be difficult.
ASU	Red	$34,400	3	$8,600	Allen	Need to balance cost savings against possible lost revenues.
ASU/main operating room	Yellow	$1,196,000	4	$398,667	Paula	The additional cases should close the remaining productivity gap.
Totals		$1,458,400		$571,400		

Note: ASU = ambulatory surgery unit; CM = contribution margin; FTE = full-time equivalent; FY = fiscal year; LOS = length of stay; PACU = post-acute care unit.

11.5), a designation of "10" under the "Current FY Months" column indicates that the accrued savings will occur for 10 of the 12 months of the current fiscal year; therefore, the risk-rated budget year cash impact for the first initiative is ten-twelfths of the annualized risk-rated opportunity.

Using the tracking template and sizing methodology, the sub-teams identify opportunities and present them to the core productivity team. The productivity team reviews each initiative in terms of validity, size, and risk and tests any assumptions made by the subteam. By the fifth meeting, the productivity team analyst should be preparing a consolidated tracking of opportunities across all the subteams.

Enablers

Some recommended improvements warrant additional investments. Collaborative teams must identify enabling investments and their associated costs. Enablers are small investments that facilitate work redesign or implementation and may include new technology or equipment, physical facility changes, new information systems, retraining, or other areas of investment. Investments that exceed expected savings do not help achieve the team's economic goals and, in most cases, should be avoided.

CASE EXAMPLE: PERFORMANCE IMPROVEMENT PLAN FOR PHARMACY SERVICES

Sheri is the director of pharmacy services for a four-hospital regional health system. She served as director for the flagship hospital until two months ago, when the system's executive team promoted her to a regional director position with responsibility for pharmacy operations across the system.

The four hospitals have been part of the same system for more than six years but have not pursued operational integration except in patient accounts and a few administrative functions. Facing reimbursement and competitive pressures, the system must reduce operating expenses to maintain a sufficient operating margin. Over the past six months, the executive staff have restructured department-level leadership positions to create regional roles in clinical and administrative functions. In establishing these new roles, system leaders seek to empower regional leaders such as Sheri to reduce operating expenses and drive consistency in processes and services to patients.

Following the management restructuring, system leaders initiated a systemwide performance improvement initiative. The organization identified four primary areas of focus:

- Labor productivity
- Supply chain and nonlabor
- Inpatient throughput
- Revenue cycle

These areas were selected, in part, on the basis of the organization's performance to benchmarks, which revealed considerable improvement opportunities. The productivity team identified labor opportunities in several functional areas. For pharmacy services, the staffing variance to the 35th percentile benchmark was ten full-time equivalents (FTEs), or 9 percent of the pharmacy labor complement across the four hospitals, which represented an annual savings of $620,000.

As a result, Sheri was asked to participate in a productivity collaborative team representing pharmacy along with regional directors of other programs that indicated PI opportunities. The productivity team would be supported by subteams assigned to each functional area. Sheri would head up the pharmacy subteam. Each subteam was charged with identifying improvements that would save half of the benchmark opportunity at the 35th percentile. For Sheri's subteam, this amount calculated to $310,000.

Before forming her subteam, Sheri decided to institute some management restructuring in pharmacy services. She converted two hospital director positions to managers, taking advantage of the new regional structure. This shift was undertaken in advance of the subteam so that the new structure would be in place to drive the process. The restructuring resulted in $125,000 in savings, which could be applied to the savings target.

After attending the productivity core team kickoff, Sheri formed a pharmacy services productivity subteam. She served as the team leader and recruited a multidisciplinary team of site managers, pharmacists, pharmacy technicians, a clinical pharmacy consultant, and a nursing manager from one of the large medical units.

Using the PI framework, Sheri led the team through an exercise of brainstorming related to key questions pertaining to the ten levers that most apply to pharmacy services. This exercise, the results of which are captured in exhibit 11.6, enabled the subteam to identify, in the first meeting, those areas that produced the most opportunities.

Through subsequent meetings, the team identified and quantified several labor improvement opportunities. Using the tracking sheet (exhibit 11.7), the team recorded four interventions totaling $535,000 in annual savings. After risk rating, the adjusted opportunity was lowered to $368,000.

Exhibit 11.6: Pharmacy Subteam Idea Brainstorming

Function: Pharmacy Services

Improvement Lever	Key Question	Brainstorming Ideas
Process improvement	What processes in the department can be simplified, eliminated, or improved in a manner that reduces resource requirements and improves customer value?	Prescription order processing, drug delivery and stocking cabinets, intravenous admixture.
Facility optimization	Are there improvements we can make to the layout of our department that will improve patient flow and facilitate effective use of our resources?	Reconfigure dispensing area within main hospital.
Role design	How can we design roles and assign responsibilities in a way that will achieve improved flexibility and workload balance across our staff?	Current skill match heavy on pharmacists, light on technicians; pharmacists are exempt, making overstaffing complex.
Demand matching	How can we do a better job of scheduling our staff so we effectively meet variable workload demand?	Decrease all staff pharmacist positions by 10% to 0.9 FTE.
Structural process improvement	What key multidepartmental and cross-entity processes can be simplified, eliminated, or improved in ways that reduce resource demand while improving value to customers?	Clinical review and consultation; working with Frontier Cancer Center to streamline outpatient chemotherapy process.
Management restructuring	Are there opportunities to leverage executive or management roles across departments, programs, and sites?	Move to regional structure for pharmacy services.

(continued)

(continued from previous page)

Exhibit 11.6: Pharmacy Subteam Idea Brainstorming
Function: Pharmacy Services

Improvement Lever	Key Question	Brainstorming Ideas
Service redeployment	Are there staffing resources and services that we should physically relocate to a different area to improve service and lower costs?	Outpatient pharmacy cost center created; 24-hour service filling approximately 100 prescriptions daily had been absorbed into inpatient pharmacy cost center.
Nonlabor optimization	Are there improvements to our supply chain processes and other nonlabor expenses that will reduce staff time and lower spending on supplies, equipment, and purchased services?	Lots of opportunity to reduce drug spend—covered by nonlabor team.
Flexible staffing	What strategies can we employ to ensure we have sufficient staffing for changes in workload volumes?	Change skill mix to leverage more technology resources.
Utilization improvement	Are there opportunities to reduce unnecessary utilization of services that will reduce the cost of care while maintaining or improving outcomes?	Significant opportunity—covered by nonlabor team.

Note: FTE = full-time equivalent.

Exhibit 11.7: Pharmacy Subteam Tracking Sheet

Item	Improvement Lever	Item Description	Units of Improvement	Value per Unit of Improvement	Annualized Run-Rate Impact	Is There a Prior History of Success in This Area?	Is Completion in Our Control?	Do Skills Currently Exist to Complete?
1	Management restructuring	Redesign regional management structure for pharmacy services by converting 2 director positions to managers.	Average pay rate	$62,500 difference per FTE	$125,000	Yes	Yes	Yes
2	Process improvement	Eliminate medication reconciliation pharmacist shift. Combine duties of two technician shifts.	FTE	2 FTEs at $30,000	$60,000	Yes	Yes	Yes
3	Dynamic staffing	Convert 3 pharmacists to technician positions.	Average pay rate	$50,000 difference per FTE × 3 FTEs	$150,000	Yes	Yes	Yes
4	Dynamic staffing	Decrease all staff pharmacist positions by 10% to 0.9 FTE.	FTE	2.5 FTEs at $80,000	$200,000	Yes	No	Yes
				Totals	**$535,000**			

(continued)

(continued from previous page)

Exhibit 11.7: Pharmacy Subteam Tracking Sheet

Risk Rating	Risk-Rated Annualized Run-Rate Impact	FY Months	Risk-Rated FY Cash Impact	Assigned to	Notes
Green	$100,000	10	$83,333		This change was implemented in November.
Green	$48,000	8	$32,000		
Green	$120,000	8	$80,000		
Yellow	$100,000	9	$75,000		
Unrated	—		—		
Unrated	—		—		
Totals	**$368,000**		**$270,333**		

Note: FTE = full-time equivalent; FY = fiscal year.

CHAPTER 12

Leading Implementation

ALTHOUGH REDESIGN CAN be challenging, many organizations find implementation to be the most difficult part of performance improvement (PI). Miles (2010) identfies the following core inhibitors to successful organizational change, most of which arise during implementation:

- *Cautious management culture.* Executives, even some on the senior team, may avoid risks, protect their business areas, and try to avoid big mistakes by sticking to the "tried and true." Caution is typical, as little reward generally ensues for those who speak out with bold, new ideas. Preoccupation with incremental improvements prevails, thwarting opportunities for breakthrough results.
- *Business-as-usual management process.* Day-to-day processes and meetings, as well as management bandwidth, are already overtaxed, and little accommodation is made for new or different approaches. Executives are therefore stuck waiting for the perfect new business model.
- *Initiative gridlock.* Frequently, too many separate initiatives are thrown at the organization and its people all at once. Uncoordinated functional initiatives, layered one on top of another, can create task overload across the hospital.
- *Recalcitrant executives.* Some executives remain unconvinced and uncommitted to the organization's

transformation agenda. They are able to avoid conflict while exhibiting an unwillingness to reallocate their resources to support the transformative agenda. Turnover at the senior level can be disruptive, but a practice of protracted tolerance of nonaligned leaders throughout the organization must be ended.

- *Disengaged employees.* The lack of understanding surrounding the need for transformation prohibits employees from grasping the new strategy and transformative agenda. Employees are not certain they will be rewarded for demonstrating the new expected behaviors and therefore do not feel safe in sharing their best ideas.
- *Loss of focus during execution.* Just when the change effort seems to be working, the process hits a slump often caused by the desire to relax immediately following the launch of new initiatives or by the daily emergencies that crop up in any business. The belief that improvements are progressing blinds executives and encourages them to take their foot off the gas.

Myriad reasons help explain the emergence of such inhibitors to successful change initiatives in organizations:

- Up to this point, change has only occurred on paper. Implementation is where change begins to involve and affect people and operations. Resistance to change is often highest at the initial stages of implementation and must be addressed proactively.
- Implementation requires more leadership time and attention than redesign requires. Leaders often must institute new processes and systems while continuing to manage day-to-day operations.
- Compared with the redesign process, implementation is protracted. Keeping focus and enthusiasm elevated over a long period can be challenging for leaders and staff involved in the process.

- Implementation requires the discipline of project management, performance measurement, change management, and organizational communications. Gaps in any of these capabilities can work against successful implementation.

For these reasons, organizations need to approach implementation with the same degree of discipline and structure that occurs during redesign.

STEERING COMMITTEE PRESENTATION AND REVIEW

Once the listing and sizing of opportunities are completed and consolidated across the subteams, each collaborative team develops a draft implementation plan. This plan informs the executive committee of the scope of the effort and time frame required for implementing proposed changes.

A standardized template is necessary to ensure implementation consistency across numerous functional areas. Exhibit 12.1 is an example of an implementation planning template for a surgery productivity team. Each line item in the tracking template corresponds with a row in the implementation template. In general, an implementation plan provides the following:

- A descriptive summary of the proposed changes or improvements
- Sequential action steps required to implement each change
- Identification of individuals responsible for completing each step
- A target completion date for each step
- When applicable, identification of the metric used to track progress and results for each intervention

Exhibit 12.1: Example of a Collaborative Team Implementation Plan for Surgical Services

Surgery Department Productivity Implementation Plan

Category/ Team	Operational Change	Action Steps	Responsibility	Completion Date	Performance Metrics	Notes
Surgery productivity team	1 supervisor position on day shift will be vacant as of 4/11. We will not fill this position.	1. Communicate design and plan to staff.	OR director	30-Mar	OR staff hours per case (productivity monitoring)	
		2. Work with supervisor team to reassign responsibilities.	Director/ supervisors	4-Apr		
		3. Conduct exit interview with outgoing supervisor.	OR director	11-Apr		
		4. Begin new supervisor schedule.	Supervisors	13-Apr		
		5. Obtain staff feedback and adjust operations accordingly.	Supervisors/staff	31-May		
Surgery productivity team	Improve throughput in PACU; reduce PACU LOS by 20%.	1. Complete throughput project with nursing.	PACU LOS team	15-Apr	Average LOS in PACU	Actual staffing reductions are contingent on how quickly the LOS can be reduced.
		2. Implement process changes.	PACU manager and staff	1-May		
		3. Monitor results and adjust staffing based on throughput improvement.	PACU manager	15-May		

(continued)

(continued from previous page)

Exhibit 12.1: Example of a Collaborative Team Implementation Plan for Surgical Services

Surgery Department Productivity Implementation Plan

Category/ Team	Operational Change	Action Steps	Responsibility	Completion Date	Performance Metrics	Notes
Surgery productivity team	Reconfigure block scheduling for orthopedic and spine cases to better balance cases across the week.	1. Finalize new blocks with orthopedic group.	Orthopedics manager	21-Apr	Block utilization %, ortho-pedic case volumes	Target utilization: 85%
		2. Get approval from block committee for go-ahead.	OR director	5-May		
		3. Implement new block and team schedule.	Orthopedics manager	1-Jun		
		4. Follow up with orthopedic surgeons on issues that arise.	Orthopedics manager/surgeons	Ongoing		
Surgery productivity team	Eliminate Saturday schedule in ASU.	1. Complete transition plan.	ASU manager	15-Apr	Case volumes	
		2. Communicate with physicians and staff.	OR director/ASU manager	30-Apr		
		3. Transition plan for affected staff.	ASU manager	15-Jun		
		4. Implement plan.	ASU manager	1-Jul		
		5. Monitor results.	OR director/ASU manager	Ongoing		

(continued)

(continued from previous page)

Exhibit 12.1: Example of a Collaborative Team Implementation Plan for Surgical Services

Surgery Department Productivity Implementation Plan

Category/ Team	Operational Change	Action Steps	Responsibility	Completion Date	Performance Metrics	Notes
Surgery productivity team	New general surgeons are expected to bring in 20 additional cases per week starting 5/1.	1. Orient new surgeons.	In-service education	1-May	Caseload for new surgeons	
		2. Finalize block assignments.	OR director	5-May		
		3. Implement plan.	OR director	15-May		
		4. Monitor results.	OR director	Ongoing		

Key performance metrics: financial, operational, customer, and human resources.

Note: ASU = ambulatory surgery unit; LOS = length of stay; OR = operating room; PACU = post-acute care unit.

An initial draft implementation plan is included as part of the steering committee presentation.

Steering Committee Presentation

As a starting point for implementation, the committee should receive a high-level summary of the opportunities identified by all the collaborative teams to determine if the overall target has been met. Exhibit 12.2 is an example of an opportunity summary for the work of seven collaborative teams. These groups identified and sized 208 improvement opportunities with a total annual economic opportunity of $39 million. After risk rating each item, the opportunity was reduced to $18.8 million. Because the organization was already several months into the new fiscal year, the amount that was achievable in the remaining year was further reduced.

The steering committee next reviews a prioritized list of opportunities for each team. These opportunities are typically presented by each team leader, but the presentation can involve other team members.

Depending on the number of collaborative teams, the steering committee may be presented with several hundred initiatives to evaluate. Because the review of all the initiatives is impossible to complete in a single meeting, opportunities should be prioritized. As shown in exhibit 12.3, prioritization should be based on the impact size and implementation difficulty. Large opportunities with relatively low implementation risk should be prioritized and approved first. The steering committee should also review large opportunities with high risk to understand the factors that will make implementation difficult.

For each opportunity reviewed, the steering committee should answer the following questions:

- Is the annualized benefit reasonable? Highly conservative estimates can underrepresent true opportunity, whereas

Exhibit 12.2: Opportunity Summary

	Items	Undiscounted Annualized Run-Rate Impact	Discounted Annualized Run-Rate Impact	Discounted Fiscal Year Impact
Customer service	17	—	—	—
Portfolio	24	$4,227,000	$2,981,100	$1,301,325
Productivity	33	$9,770,857	$4,783,373	$2,908,125
Revenue cycle	21	$3,419,906	$1,984,978	$1,073,422
Supply chain	40	$4,679,874	$2,825,299	$1,249,967
Tactical growth	54	$16,033,130	$5,663,770	$1,299,877
Throughput	19	$881,250	$585,750	$195,250
Total	208	$39,012,017	$18,824,270	$8,027,966

Effect of risk rating: $(20,187,746)

Effect of implementation rating: $(10,796,305)

Exhibit 12.3: Prioritization Framework

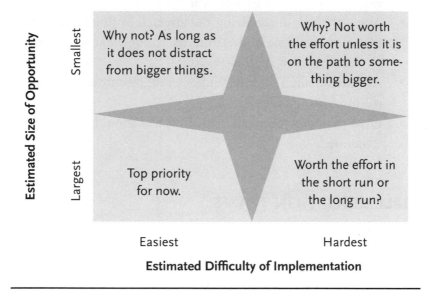

Estimated Size of Opportunity

Smallest — Why not? As long as it does not distract from bigger things.

Smallest — Why? Not worth the effort unless it is on the path to something bigger.

Largest — Top priority for now.

Largest — Worth the effort in the short run or the long run?

Easiest   Hardest

Estimated Difficulty of Implementation

overstating the impact can jeopardize achievement of the target.

- Is the risk rating appropriate? Similar issues occur with under- or overestimating the implementation risks.
- Will implementing this item distract from success with other, larger initiatives?
- Can additional resources or administrative support reduce the risk level of high-risk opportunities?
- Is the estimated time for implementation correct? Can implementation occur earlier for critical opportunities?
- Which initiatives, if any, should be deferred or not pursued?

Once the steering committee has fully vetted the list of priority initiatives, attention should turn to implementation planning. In this phase, senior leaders should perform the following tasks:

- Review the draft implementation plans for major initiatives and determine if the approach, timing, and assigned responsibilities are correct.
- Assess the risk in achieving the targeted improvements in the estimated time frame, and determine what actions can be taken to mitigate these risks.
- Access and align internal and external resources necessary to support implementation.
- Determine how implementation teams should be structured.

IMPLEMENTATION TEAMS

Like redesign, implementation is primarily performed by multidisciplinary teams with assigned responsibilities and deadlines. Implementation teams do not necessarily adopt the same structure as collaborative teams. Considering no set rules dictate the size and number of implementation teams, some organizations assign small implementation teams to a few initiatives. This approach requires the coordination of a large number of teams, but it engages more staff and can expedite implementation.

The work of one collaborative team may require multiple implementation teams. For example, as shown in exhibit 12.4, a throughput collaborative team designed implementation plans for subteams focused on the three areas of redesign: transition and discharge, intensive care unit (ICU) throughput, and bed management.

Implementation teams include members of the original collaborative team and may engage others as well, including staff who are most significantly affected by the redesign. The duration and number of implementation team meetings depend largely on the tasks assigned to a team. For some, implementation may occur over several weeks, while complex changes take six months or longer.

Exhibit 12.4: Example of Implementation Teams for Improving Throughput

Throughput Implementation Teams		Patient Day Reduction	Risk-Rated Annual Run Rate
Transition/discharge	➡	3,400	$425,500
ICU throughput	➡	470	$56,400
Bed management	➡	350	$43,800
Totals:		4,220	$525,700
	FY impact:		$195,200

Note: FY = fiscal year; ICU = intensive care unit.

Implementation teams take on numerous responsibilities. To help teams manage these duties, prior to implementing any changes, steering committee leaders should

- communicate the details of the approved redesign tasks to staff and other stakeholders;
- approve the final draft of the implementation plan for tasks assigned to the team;
- secure the necessary PI, information technology, and similar resources to support implementation;
- confirm and finalize performance metrics and the processes for ongoing measurement; and
- provide communication and support to team members and other affected staff.

Team leaders are responsible for keeping implementation members focused on the task at hand. Implementation teams should not be a forum for continued debate on the merits of proposed solutions or for generating design alternatives.

During implementation, teams are responsible for the following:

- *Leading the launch.* Team leaders and members implement operational changes approved by the steering committee in accordance with the implementation plan.
- *Coaching staff during the transition.* Team leaders and members serve as the internal champions of the changes and, as such, are responsible for selling the changes in the organization and bringing others along in the process.
- *Fielding questions and soliciting feedback from staff.* Questions arise from staff who are not part of the implementation team but are affected by the redesign. Team members should be held accountable for providing clear and consistent answers. Staff should also have a means for providing feedback throughout the implementation period.
- *Piloting results and adjusting the design accordingly.* Frequently, unanticipated modifications to initial redesign plans arise. Some of these alterations are necessary and beneficial. Leaders must be able to discern needed alterations to the plan that still achieve the target and do not undermine the principles of the redesign.
- *Monitoring performance metrics.* Measuring the effectiveness of implementation depends on measuring performance. Implementation teams must use data to establish performance baselines and monitor performance after implementation.

Implementation teams vary in size, duration, and focus depending on the nature of the redesign. Team membership and timelines should reflect the type and level of effort required to complete the transition. As shown in exhibit 12.5, some improvement levers correspond to relatively short-term, straightforward implementation, while others take considerably more time and effort. A radiology director, for example, can implement new staffing schedules in a few weeks to improve labor demand matching. This type of change can occur without forming an implementation team. In contrast, a portfolio change, such as adding a service or outsourcing an existing function, can take considerable time and involve numerous leaders and staff.

Organizing and deploying implementation teams require the attention and forethought of leaders. The following case study is an example of how one health system constructed implementation teams and aligned specific improvement initiatives.

Exhibit 12.5: Implementation Characteristics of Improvement Levers

Improvement Category	Improvement Levers	Typical Implementation Characteristics
Improving processes and facilities	• Process improvement • Structural process improvement • Physical reconfiguration	• Shorter implementation schedule • Much longer facility modification time frame, depending on the extent of the redesign • Possible need for piloting and adjusting to process changes • Need for multidisciplinary team, particularly for cross-functional processes • Need for staff training on new processes
Aligning resources with demand	• Role and team redesign • Demand smoothing • Dynamic staffing • Demand regrouping	• Shorter implementation schedule • Possible need for staff training and development • Ability for some changes to be implemented by department leaders without the need for a full implementation team • Longer implementation time for team design in patient care

(continued)

(continued from previous page)

Exhibit 12.5: Implementation Characteristics of Improvement Levers

Improvement Category	Improvement Levers	Typical Implementation Characteristics
Leveraging the system	• Management restructuring • System rationalization • Service redeployment	• Longer implementation time frame (6 weeks or greater) due to complexities of multisite coordination • Possible impact of severance policies on timing and cost savings of management restructuring • Need for process redesign in service redeployment; requires multidisciplinary team to implement
Optimizing nonlabor expenses	• Nonlabor optimization	• Impact of purchasing contract changes on implementation timing • Quick occurrence of some supply changes in commodity and routine supplies • Much longer implementation time requirement for producer price index product changes • Possible impact from contractual requirements on purchased services changes
Improving quality and outcomes	• Utilization improvement • Off-quality improvement	• Long implementation timeline for utilization and quality changes • Requirement of multidisciplinary teams with significant involvement of physicians and clinical staff • Benefit accrual over a long time frame
Optimizing the service portfolio	• Service outsourcing • Service divestment • Continuum realignment	• Need for long-term implementation and planning for portfolio decisions • Possible requirement of extensive leadership communication and support for affected employees • Possible need for involvement of external partnering organizations for implementation
Building top-line revenues	• Demand growth • Revenue optimization	• Possible inclusion of both short-term, tactical interventions and long-term growth strategies for growth to occur • Short-term process changes and retraining required for revenue cycle improvement

CASE EXAMPLE: ORGANIZING FOR IMPLEMENTATION

A regional health system completed a transformation project to close a financial gap and improve margin performance. During the design phase, the organization deployed six collaborative teams focused on the following areas:

- Clinical utilization
- Nonlabor
- Productivity and workforce management
- Throughput
- Revenue cycle
- Growth

The collaborative teams included representatives from the system's entities, including three hospitals, a physician services division, and a corporate services office. Several of the collaborative teams used subteams representing individual entities or service lines. Collectively, the teams produced more than 140 improvement initiatives with a total risk-rated annual impact of $25 million. Included in these opportunities were small, entity-specific initiatives; broad, system-level interventions; and initiatives pertaining to specific service lines.

The steering committee next needed to determine how to organize and assign these initiatives to implementation teams. First, the group identified current teams and committees that could assume implementation responsibilities. For example, the organization operated standing committees for managing key service lines. The steering committee grouped initiatives according to service line, including orthopedics, cardiac surgery, and neurosurgery, and assigned these to the service line committees. These groups assumed responsibility for implementing initiatives pertaining to length of stay, cost per case utilization improvement, and related supply savings.

Some initiatives were assigned to system-level teams. Many supply chain initiatives were assigned to a system-level implementation team, as control for achieving most of these savings (e.g., pricing and other contract changes) resided with the system-level materials management group. Other initiatives involving productivity and nonlabor improvement were assigned to site-specific teams, as execution and management of these projects rested largely with site-based leadership.

Exhibit 12.6 provides a partial list of the implementation teams identified and chartered by the steering committee. In all, the organization deployed 36 teams to drive implementation for the 142 initiatives.

ADDRESSING IMPLEMENTATION ISSUES

Collaborative teams identify, at a high level, redesign opportunities for improving operational performance. Implementation teams are responsible for addressing the detailed process issues required to operationalize the changes. For this reason, implementation teams routinely confront unexpected issues and previously unanticipated details that must be addressed before finalizing the design.

Modifications to the intended design should be approached carefully. Before changes are adopted, implementation teams should first review the original design criteria and principles used by the responsible collaborative team. Small alterations that maintain the integrity of the intended design may proceed without executive approval. However, changes that violate the intended design tenets should be reviewed and approved by the steering committee. Frequently, design changes result from implementation difficulties such as staff or leader resistance. The steering committee must differentiate these instances from cases in which a major design change is justifiable.

Implementation teams need to track each issue and determine the best resolution. Exhibit 12.7 is an example of an issue tracking sheet for an emergency department implementation team. After piloting a flexible staffing plan, the implementation team identified several process issues to address. This template was used in the team meetings to capture each issue, identify potential solutions, and assign responsibilities.

After Implementation

The work of the implementation team concludes when all the initiatives under their scope have been implemented and are performing to target. Performance metrics are monitored by functional-area leaders to ensure that processes remain in control. For large-scale changes, implementation teams should reconvene periodically over the next year to discuss any issues and redesign considerations.

Project Management Office

Large implementation initiatives tend to achieve better outcomes when they are supported by project management staffing and systems than when such support is absent. Many organizations establish a project management office (PMO) to support the work of multiple implementation teams. PMOs are central resource areas that provide technical design and implementation assistance. PMO staff members are usually internal staff with proficiencies in the following:

- PI tools and concepts
- Information systems and analytics
- Change management
- Organizational communications

Exhibit 12.6: Example of a Collaborative Implementation Team Summary

Team No.	Implementation Team	Initiative No.	Original Collaborative Team	Initiative Title	Risk-Rated Annual Impact by Entity					Grand Total
					Hospital A	Hospital B	Hospital C	Physician Division	Corporate Services	
11	Pharmaceutical team—system	97, 98, 99	Nonlabor	Formulary changes and drug repricing—pharmacy	$779,000	$137,300	$199,400			$1,115,700
12	Physician services—growth team	25, 26, 27	Growth	Reduced leakage from physician network practices	$3,261,647	$875,768	$372,214			$4,509,629
13	Physician services—revenue cycle team	18–22	Revenue cycle	Improved professional documentation and coding				$1,230,000		$1,230,000
		23	Revenue cycle	Improved POS collections				$550,000		$550,000
15	Hospital OP growth team	28, 29, 30	Growth	Outpatient services growth initiatives	$350,000	$275,000	$210,000			$835,000
17	Reprocessing team—system	34, 35, 36	Nonlabor	System supply chain—purchased services	$329,100	$42,600	$62,800			$434,500
21	Revenue cycle team—system	60, 61	Revenue cycle	Improved professional documentation and coding	$446,000	$315,500				$761,500
		63, 64		Improved POS collections	$415,300	$207,000				$622,300
24	Supply chain team—system	41, 42, 43	Nonlabor	System supply chain—supplies—medical–surgical	$550,700	$71,400	$105,100			$727,200
		51, 52, 53	Nonlabor	System supply chain—supplies—other		$5,100	$4,600			$9,700
		37, 38, 39	Nonlabor	System supply chain—supplies—standardization	$235,600	$30,500	$44,900			$311,000

(continued)

(*continued from previous page*)

Exhibit 12.6: Example of a Collaborative Implementation Team Summary

Team No.	Implementation Team	Initiative No.	Original Collaborative Team	Initiative Title	Risk-Rated Annual Impact by Entity						Grand Total
					Hospital A	Hospital B	Hospital C	Physician Division	Corporate Services		
25	Productivity and nonlabor team—corporate services	134, 135, 136	Productivity	Span-of-control reductions					$215,000		$215,000
		66	Nonlabor	Reductions in budgeted nonlabor expenses					$12,500		$12,500
28	Productivity team—hospital A	131, 132, 133	Productivity	Departmental productivity targets	$355,000						$355,000
29	OR throughput team—hospital A	79	Throughput	Lower perioperative LOS	$124,000						$124,000
30	OR throughput team—hospital B	80	Throughput	Lower perioperative LOS		$144,700					$144,700
											$16,735,542

Note: LOS = length of stay; OP = outpatient; OR = operating room; POS = point of service.

Exhibit 12.7: Implementation Issues Tracking Document

Emergency Department Implementation Issues
Updated: 3/22

Issue	Description	Solution	Follow-Up
Intake process	The function of the intake staff is not defined under staffing plan B.	Develop protocols and roles for how intake staff are utilized under plan B.	Implement revised protocols on 4/1; communicate with staff at 3/28 department meeting.
Staffing plan switch (plan A to plan B)	The process is not well defined for when to switch from staffing plan A to plan B.	Develop comprehensive criteria for when department converts from plan A to plan B.	3/20: New criteria developed; need to communicate to staff and run trial before 4/1; need to include the use of overflow beds in standard process.
Case management (CM) early warning	Early warning protocols are not being used uniformly by case managers to alert the units.	Meet with CM staff and retrain; continue to audit individual performance.	*Not scheduled*—need to assign lead.
Capacity management	Night shift frequently fails to close zone A despite low census after midnight. The department needs criteria defined on when to close east zone.	Develop conditional criteria for 7:00 p.m.–7:00 a.m. shift staff and communicate.	3/17: Communicated to night manager defined criteria and staff drawdown protocols. Will continue to monitor.
Telephone routing	The unit clerks do not consistently route incoming calls to the emergency department (ED).	Develop routing procedures for inbound calls to the ED.	3/21: Seems to be more prevalent on day shift; meet with staff to identify root causes.
Patient egress	The checkout process is broken; too many patients leave without checking out. As a result, we are not meeting our point-of-service collection targets.	Assign a team to review processes and develop recommendations— need by 4/1.	3/13: Team kickoff event takes place. 3/15: Implement quick-win ideas to improve process. 3/29: Report-out scheduled.
Registration staff orientation	New registration staff often do not understand the ED contingency staffing plan.	Schedule orientation for staff; need several sessions for days/nights/ weekends.	3/21: Need to schedule with patient access—director has been on vacation.
Metrics transparency	Need a way to communicate patient volume, back-log, etc., in real time to staff. This process will help staff anticipate change in staffing plan.	Implementation team to meet with the information technology department to research.	Schedule meeting.

During the implementation phase, PMO staff undertake the following:

- Establish standard processes and systems for implementation management.
- Create a central point for the gathering and reporting of performance metrics.
- Help teams define clear goals and create effective work plans.
- Educate and train team leaders on project leadership skills.
- Assist with piloting and process revisions that occur during implementation.
- Capture lessons learned for improvements with future projects.
- Leverage management systems for project management and performance tracking.
- Provide structured and consistent status reporting to the senior leadership team.

Successful implementation requires organizational discipline to keep leaders and staff focused on execution. Staffing resources, project management tools, and technical expertise must be available to support staff who are driving implementation. Executives must provide persistent leadership and hold managers accountable for results. Most important, leaders must sell the organization on the benefits of redesign, address resistance to change, and remove implementation barriers.

CHAPTER 13

Three Disciplines for Holding the Gains

OFTEN, HEALTHCARE ORGANIZATIONS successfully redesign and implement operational improvements only to lose the gains over ensuing years. Leadership changes, market dynamics, organizational inertia, and other factors slowly erode performance advancements. High-performing health systems institute and adhere to organizational disciplines that help retain performance improvement (PI) gains. While many factors contribute to long-term improvement success, three disciplines are vital for keeping organizations on track with their PI initiatives:

- A comprehensive system to continuously manage labor performance
- An ongoing process and structure to evaluate supplies and other nonlabor resources
- A structured process to continuously manage the organization's service portfolio and growth opportunities

LABOR PERFORMANCE MANAGEMENT SYSTEM

Effective health systems manage labor productivity through the execution of thoughtful planning, consistent measurement and monitoring, and continuous improvement. Supporting these disciplines are the requisite information systems, processes, and policies of an effective labor management system.

A labor productivity management system (exhibit 13.1) consists of four essential components:

- *Budgeting and forecasting*, to set baselines and expectations of future performance
- *Position control*, to continuously regulate the balance of labor resources with changing workload demand
- *Benchmarking*, to establish performance standards and identify high-performing practices
- *Productivity monitoring*, to measure and evaluate actual versus planned labor performance over time

Deficiencies in one or more of these components limit an organization's ability to achieve productivity performance goals and control labor expenses.

Exhibit 13.1: Labor Performance Management System

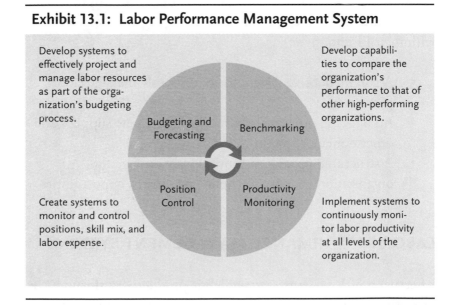

328   *18 Levers for High-Impact Performance Improvement*

Labor Forecasting and Budgeting

Annual budgeting is a common process in healthcare organizations. Operating budgets serve the following purposes:

- Anticipating and planning for changes in workload volumes
- Allocating limited resources and investment across numerous business units and programs
- Identifying and planning capital investments
- Setting performance standards and goals for leaders
- Ensuring investments are aligned with the organization's strategic priorities

Most healthcare organizations adopt an annual fixed budget for labor, supplies, and other operating expenses. Typically, the budget is based on the previous year's actual spending and adjusted for expected volume changes, inflation, productivity assumptions, and other factors. Once developed and approved, the fixed budget usually remains unaltered over the course of the fiscal year.

Some healthcare organizations utilize a variable budget. This approach adjusts departmental budgeted expenses on the basis of actual workload volumes. A variable budgeting approach can be beneficial in instances where workload rapidly changes (up or down) or is unpredictable.

Labor comprises the majority of a hospital's operating expenses and, as such, should be scrutinized during the budget development process. Labor budgeting should be a collaborative process engaging leaders throughout the organization. Budgets prepared in a top-down manner frequently lack buy-in from department directors and middle managers, leading to difficulties in holding leaders accountable.

Although no single best method for budget development exists, the following basic practices are highly effective for most organizations:

- Budgeted labor hours and costs are derived from forecasted workload volumes. Fixed and variable staff designations are made at the job-class level and applied to the forecasts.
- Premium pay use, including overtime, is evaluated and projected by job class as part of the budgeting process.
- Merit-pay and cost-of-living adjustments are factored into the budget at the job-class level on the basis of when adjustments take effect during the year.
- Patient care staffing is determined by defined staffing matrixes that are reflected in the department's labor budget. Matrixes are built on the basis of engineered standards and account for acuity differences across units.
- The organization employs multiple hospitalwide labor productivity metrics (e.g., full-time equivalents [FTEs] per adjusted admission, labor expense as a percentage of net revenues) and goals to establish overall targets for labor budgeting.
- In cases of budgetary increases in staffing, managers are uniformly required to provide supporting evidence to justify increased staffing.

The process of developing a labor budget (exhibit 13.2) begins with establishing and projecting a department's units of service (UOS). Each cost center should have a primary UOS for measuring workload. Ideally, the same UOS should be used to drive a department's operating budget, productivity monitoring system, and benchmarking. In variable patient care areas, the UOS is usually a count of charge transactions that correspond to the number of tests, procedures, or cases performed over time. Tying the UOS to a chargeable transaction reduces the need for manual workload reporting and helps eliminate the inaccuracies that can occur with manual reporting.

Fixed departments, such as administration, staff education, and the medical staff office, should also have an assigned UOS. These

Exhibit 13.2: Labor Budget Development Process

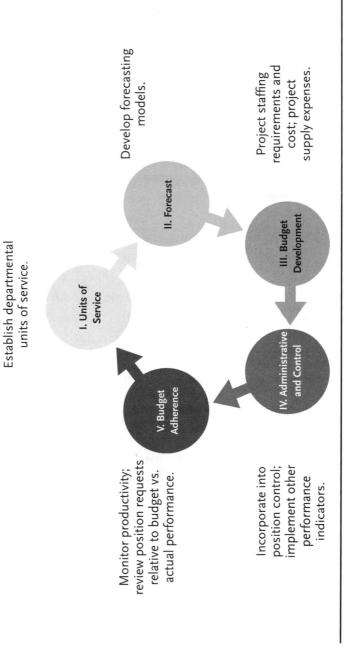

Establish departmental
units of service.

Develop forecasting
models.

Project staffing
requirements and
cost; project
supply expenses.

I. Units of
Service

II. Forecast

III. Budget
Development

IV. Administrative
and Control

V. Budget
Adherence

Monitor productivity;
review position requests
relative to budget vs.
actual performance.

Incorporate into
position control;
implement other
performance
indicators.

areas should be given an organization-wide workload indicator, such as adjusted discharges or total patient days. This practice ensures that fixed overhead costs are managed in accordance with the organization's overall workload trends (and their associated revenues).

A *departmental operating budget* should be built on a forecast of the total units of service anticipated for the next budget year. The forecasting model should estimate high-level organizational volumes as follows:

- Inpatient discharges and patient days by service line
- Outpatient and emergency department visits by program
- Ambulatory visits for physician services and other non-acute services

Workload forecasts should reflect the organization's strategic planning goals and service line objectives for the coming year. If, for example, the orthopedic service line expects to grow joint replacement surgeries by 10 percent in the coming year, the increase should be reflected in workload forecasts for all areas affected—including nursing, surgery, materials management, laboratory, and rehabilitative services, among others.

Forecasts should also account for anticipated savings resulting from current or future improvement initiatives. For example, if the hospital expects to improve overall length of stay by 5 percent, this reduction should be factored into forecasted patient days. Hardwiring future improvements into the operating budget is a critical component for ensuring that leaders effectively implement planned improvement opportunities.

Departmental Labor Budgets

Operating budgets are created by projecting costs for each general ledger (G/L) account in each cost center. G/L accounts should be designated appropriately to provide sufficient detail of labor expenses. Typically, hospitals break out labor expenses into several categories, including the following:

- Salary and wages
- Overtime and premium pay
- Paid time off
- Bonuses
- FICA (Federal Insurance Contributions Act–mandated withholdings)
- Other pay

These accounts should be quantified at either the job-code level or by broader labor categories (e.g., management, professional, technical, clerical). Agency and contract labor usage should also be included in the operating budget and held to the same scrutiny as payroll staffing.

In addition to quantifying labor dollars, departmental labor budgets should define authorized staffing levels (productive and paid FTEs) by cost center at the job-code level. This information is commonly called a table of organization (TO) report. Each manager should have an approved TO to develop new staff schedules, design recruitment plans, and identify other required staffing adjustments. With the start of the new fiscal year, the organization's position control report should be updated to reflect the new authorized staffing levels.

Budget Administration and Control

The monthly budget report is a primary tool for managing operational performance at the department level and across the business enterprise. Managers need effective reporting systems that accurately reflect cost and revenue performance and allow them to compare that performance to expectations. Labor performance budget reporting should be characterized by the following, at a minimum:

- Managers receive timely, detailed reports comparing budgeted to actual labor usage on a monthly basis. Reports show month and fiscal year to date (FYTD) variances. Comparisons are made to the same period the previous year.
- Managers are provided detailed budgeted versus actual expenses for each pay category (as opposed to a single line

item for labor expenses). Data are provided to show pay category usage by job class.

- Managers are well versed in departmental budgets and reporting. Finance provides timely, ongoing support and training to managers and assists leaders in budget development, midyear budget adjustments, and other support.
- Senior managers are provided roll-up reports showing budgeted to actual FTEs and costs by department each pay period. FYTD and trending information are also tracked. Additionally, overall FTEs and costs are tracked biweekly at the division and organization-wide levels.
- When required, the organization amends budgets during the year to reflect significant reductions or additions that occur in a department.

Budget Adherence

Budget accountability is often a defining dimension of an organization's leadership culture. High-performing organizations hold all leaders accountable for keeping expenses within budgeted levels. These organizations typically require managers to provide written justification when budget variances occur.

Even when a fixed budget is used, a department's budget performance should be evaluated relative to the volume of work performed. Labor expenses should be under budget in areas where actual workload is tracking below budgeted volumes. Similarly, departments with workload exceeding budgeted volumes should justify additional staffing and expense required to accommodate the added volume.

Position Control Systems

The workforce requirements of a health system continuously evolve. During the year, new programs and services are initiated, requiring additional staffing and new skills. Other programs are scaled back or eliminated, necessitating staffing redeployment and reductions. Demand variation, due to seasonality and other factors, can quickly accelerate or reduce staffing needs in acute care and other patient care services.

For these and other reasons, healthcare leaders need effective position control systems in place to continuously balance the supply of available staffing with the demand for services. Position control systems should work in tandem with the operating budget and productivity monitoring systems. While productivity monitoring helps leaders assess and assign staffing on a daily basis, position control systems support periodic staffing decisions pertaining to new positions and replacing recently vacated positions. Position control systems include three key components:

- Position control reporting
- A standardized staffing requisition process
- Position evaluation and control

Position Control Reporting

Managers with staffing responsibilities need consistently updated information about actual staffing and how usage compares to authorized levels. Standard budget reports typically provide monthly comparisons of budgeted to actual labor dollars expended. Although this information has value, it does not provide the necessary level of detail to support ongoing staffing decisions. Similarly, position control committees need current information on actual and authorized staffing for evaluating new position requests and refilling vacant, authorized positions.

Exhibit 13.3 provides an example of a standard position control report for healthcare organizations. At a minimum, a position control report should encompass the following attributes:

- *Frequency.* A position control report should be available to managers at least biweekly, usually corresponding to the payroll period.

Exhibit 13.3: Example of a Position Control Report

Position Control Report
Payroll Ending: 09/02/09
Department: 3 West (cost center 345)

Job Class	Job Title	Employee Name	Scheduled Hours	Regular Hours	Overtime Hours	Productive Hours	Nonproductive Hours	Paid Hours	Authorized Hours	Variance from Authorized
010	Unit manager	Thompson, Bette	80	64	0	64	16	80	80	0
Total for job class			**80**	**64**	**0**	**64**	**16**	**80**	**80**	
015	Registered nurse	Walker, Roger	80	80	8	88	0	88		
		Smithers, Cyndi	80	64	0	64	16	80		
		Wright, Carrie	40	40	0	40	0	40		
		Faldwell, Lyn	80	62	2	64	16	80		
		Mielder, Kimberly	80	64	0	64	16	80		
		Pohling, Erin	40	32	0	32	8	40		
		Fuchs, Belinda	0	32	0	32	0	32		
		Woodard, Salie	0	16	0	16	0	16		
		Best, Cindy	80	80	8	88	0	88		
		Haroldson, Pauline	80	40	0	40	40	80		

(continued)

(continued from previous page)

Exhibit 13.3: Example of a Position Control Report

Position Control Report
Payroll Ending: 09/02/09
Department: 3 West (cost center 345)

Job Class	Job Title	Employee Name	Scheduled Hours	Regular Hours	Overtime Hours	Productive Hours	Nonproductive Hours	Paid Hours	Authorized Hours	Variance from Authorized
		Stephens, Anna	80	62	2	64	16	80		
		Mitchell, Sue	80	62	2	64	16	80		
		AGENCY	0	110	0	110	0	110		
Total for job class			**720**	**744**	**22**	**766**	**128**	**895**	**820**	**−75**
016	Patient care technician	Miles, Brenda	40	40	8	48	0	48		
		Alonzo, Susan	80	72		72	8	80		
		Kent, Nancy	80	80	2	82	0	82		
		Petersen, Amy	40	32	8	32	8	40		
		Ebert, William	40	40	8	48	0	48		
		Kister, Bryan	40	40	8	48	0	48		
		Fitzpatrick, Mike	80	72		72	8	80		

(continued)

(continued from previous page)

Exhibit 13.3: Example of a Position Control Report

Position Control Report
Payroll Ending: 09/02/09
Department: 3 West (cost center 345)

Job Class	Job Title	Employee Name	Scheduled Hours	Regular Hours	Overtime Hours	Productive Hours	Nonproductive Hours	Paid Hours	Authorized Hours	Variance from Authorized
		Henderson, Lori	32	32	2	34	0	34		
Total for job class			432	408	28	436	24	460	460	0
019	Unit secretary	Russet, Patty	80	72	0	72	8	80		
		Gonzalez, Maria	80	72	0	72	8	80		
		Hodge, Rochella	80	80	0	80	0	80		
Total for job class			240	224	0	224	16	240	160	–80
Total for department			1,472	1,440	50	1,490	184	1,675	1,520	–155
		Full-time equivalents				18.6		20.9	19.0	–1.9

- *Key data elements.* The report should provide an employee-level summary of actual versus authorized hours (productive and nonproductive) for the period. Employees should be grouped by job class, so managers can track skill-mix usage and use of hours by role category. Each employee should have an assigned number of scheduled or otherwise authorized hours. A full-time staff member, for example, would be scheduled for 80 hours in a two-week pay period.

- *As-needed and temporary staff.* Agency, temporary, and as-needed (PRN) staffing hours should be included in the position control report. Their inclusion is especially important in acute care nursing and other areas that use float and PRN personnel. Generally, PRN staff do not work a set number of authorized hours; that said, their hours worked and paid should be applied against the department's budgeted hours.

- *Authorized staffing.* The report should reflect both authorized (usually budgeted) total hours and hours by skill level, and calculate variances from actual for each reporting period. Ideally, the authorized hours field should be continuously updated to reflect budget adjustments and staffing decisions made during the year.

Standardized Staffing Requisition

A second component of a position control system is a standard process for evaluating and processing staffing requisitions. Organizations should have a clearly defined process in place for managers to follow when requesting new positions or refilling vacant positions. Managers should be instructed to support requests with data—including productivity monitoring information, benchmark comparative data, historical trending information, and current position control reports. The process should be supported by a written policy and adhered to by all managers in the organization.

Most organizations have controls for adding new positions to their system. Requesting leaders are required to provide justification in the form of growing workload volumes, potential increases to or new revenues, improved patient service levels, and other factors. The same level of scrutiny is often not applied to filling vacant, authorized positions. Managers may be held to a fixed budget that allows them to refill authorized positions without considering work volume changes and other circumstances. This level of control is adequate for organizations that are performing well financially. However, a greater level of scrutiny is needed for organizations experiencing declines in workload and revenues.

Staff turnover is a chronic problem for many healthcare organizations. High levels of staff turnover can lead to high costs associated with orienting and training new employees; reduced service for patients; and increased use of overtime, agency, and other premium-pay staffing. Despite the disadvantages, staffing turnover provides leaders with opportunities to improve performance. Too often, leaders refill an existing role without considering whether the role is still required or optimally designed for changing work requirements. Leaders should view vacated positions as an opportunity to rethink how services are provided, roles are defined, and responsibilities are distributed among staff.

Attrition management can also help organizations improve productivity and reach benchmark targets while avoiding or limiting the use of layoffs. This strategy can help minimize severance expenses and other costs (tangible and intangible) associated with layoffs.

Position Evaluation and Control

The third component of a position control system is a standardized process for position evaluation that applies consistent criteria to decision making on new and replacement position requests. Increasingly, healthcare systems charge a central position control committee with evaluating all position requests.

Typically, the position control committee membership includes the following:

- The human resources (HR) executive
- The chief operating officer, the chief nursing officer, and influential operational vice presidents
- The HR manager with primary responsibilities for staff recruitment
- The PI leader or a data analyst
- Leaders of the service lines affected by the positions at issue

Other leaders may attend position control meetings on an as-needed basis to provide input on positions they have requested or have knowledge about. Committee meetings usually occur weekly to process position requests in a timely manner.

Exhibit 13.4 is a set of criteria that can be used for evaluating position requests. Position control committees evaluate requests using information available from other components of the productivity management system as follows.

- Refilling a position:
  - Is the position budgeted or otherwise authorized?
  - Is the department currently operating within its budget?
  - Will filling the position keep the department within its labor budget?
  - Will the position maintain the skill mix that is authorized for the department?
  - Is the department's productivity monitoring performance at or above targeted levels?
  - Do external benchmarks indicate significant opportunity for the department to operate at a decreased staffing level?

- Has the work requirement changed, necessitating a change in role designation or position elimination?
- Staffing a new position:
  - Is the addition justified by increased workload?
  - Will the position result in increased revenues?
  - Will the position reduce agency and overtime usage in the department?
  - Is the need for the position temporary or ongoing?
  - Is the position, as requested, the optimal skill level required for the work?

Exhibit 13.4: Sample Criteria for Evaluating Position Requests

A. Replacing Vacant Authorized Positions

Decision Criteria	Notes
1. The department has completed all required paperwork and provided supporting information and analysis for refilling an open position.	The department should complete and send a requisition document indicating the name of the employee who is vacating the position.
2. The request is for a position and skill level that have been approved for the department's baseline budget.	The department should demonstrate that the position is within the authorized staffing for the skill level requested (see current position control report).
3. The department is currently operating at or below its targeted staff hours per unit of service according to its productivity monitoring report.	The department should show a sustained trend (4–5 pay periods) of consistently operating below targeted hours per unit of service.
4. The department should demonstrate that the staffing need is long term, as opposed to a short-term seasonal need.	If the need is short term on the basis of seasonal demand, filling the position with PRN staff, agency staff, or existing staff working overtime may be more economical.

(continued)

(continued from previous page)

Exhibit 13.4: Sample Criteria for Evaluating Position Requests

B. Adding a Position

Decision Criteria	Notes
1. The department has completed all required paperwork for filling a new position.	The department should provide the estimated cost for the position and supporting rationale for its need.
2. The department is currently operating at or below its targeted staff hours per unit of service according to its productivity monitoring report.	The department should show a sustained trend (4–5 pay periods) of consistently operating below targeted hours per unit of service.
3. The department is operating within its authorized number of FTEs in total and by skill level.	Refilling a vacant authorized position with the new position—resulting in an FTE-neutral change—may be possible.
4. The department has demonstrated that the staffing need is long term, as opposed to a short-term seasonal need.	If the need is short term on the basis of seasonal demand, filling the position with PRN staff, agency staff, or existing staff working overtime may be more economical.
5. The position will replace sustained usage of overtime, agency, and other premium-pay staff as well as call pay.	The full cost of the position (inclusive of benefits) should be compared with the projected reduction in premium and call pay.
6. The position is required for new revenue generation.	The department should prove that additional revenues will be difficult or impossible to achieve without the new position. Annual net revenues should be calculated when possible.
7. Filling the position will result in a reduction in operating expenses.	For positions that reduce operating expenses, the department should quantify savings that will be difficult or impossible to achieve without the new position.

Note: FTE = full-time equivalent; PRN = as needed.

Performance Benchmarking

Benchmarking is useful to gauge organizational performance against that of peer institutions and to identify improvement opportunities. Labor hours and expense are among the most common applications of benchmarking in the healthcare industry. Labor benchmark standards and information should be employed to support other components of the labor management system. Specifically, benchmarks should be used in the following activities:

- *Budgeting.* Organizations can use benchmark hours and cost per UOS to develop target budgets for departments and programs. Many organizations, for example, target overall productivity performance at a set percentile value (typically between the 25th and 50th percentile) across all departments.
- *Productivity monitoring.* Benchmarks should be used as the target performance level in the productivity monitoring system. Productivity monitoring enables leaders to continuously evaluate actual hours and cost per UOS compared to external benchmark targets.
- *Position control.* Benchmarks should be used as part of the criteria for evaluating new position requests and as part of the position control process for evaluating requests to refill authorized positions.

A number of healthcare benchmarking systems are available in the market. When evaluating benchmarking systems, an organization should ensure that benchmarking resources offer the following:

- A sufficient number of comparative hospitals with similar macro operating characteristics, such as annual discharges, case mix index, total revenues, and teaching or nonteaching designation

- A well-designed and well-managed process for ensuring that comparative data are gathered and reported consistently across organizations
- Labor benchmarks for all functional areas of the organization
- A breakdown of labor performance and improvement opportunity for
  - efficiency variance, or the opportunity to improve the number of hours per UOS, and
  - rate variance, or the opportunity to improve the cost per UOS (accounting for skill mix, premium pay use, and other variables that increase average hourly pay rates)
- Transparent information regarding which hospitals are included in the comparative group
- Sufficient training and support, so managers are engaged and understand the information and how to use it
- A facilitated process for linking managers with their peers at other organizations for sharing information and best practices

When first introducing benchmarks, managers need to spend time gaining an understanding of the benchmarks and making corrective adjustments to the data. Leaders should establish a deadline for completing this work and coordinating data changes with the vendor.

Executives should promulgate benchmarking as a continuing process for identifying improvement opportunities. In addition to comparative data, benchmarking should include surveying and sharing high-performance practices with peer organizations.

Productivity Monitoring

Effective labor management requires information systems to monitor productivity performance on a continuous basis. Productivity monitoring systems track the labor expended in a department relative to the volume of work performed. Two primary data sources drive productivity monitoring: payroll data on hours worked and paid, and workload totals for the reporting period. Ideally, productivity monitoring workload indicators are the same UOS metrics used in departmental benchmarking and budgeting.

The productivity monitoring system should provide timely information on how well a department matches labor resources to workload demand. Many organizations produce productivity reports every two weeks to correspond to the payroll period. Although beneficial, a two-week lag can impede a leader's ability to quickly identify and correct low productivity performance. High-performing organizations use daily productivity monitoring to facilitate immediate staffing decisions and adjustments.

A labor productivity monitoring system should provide the following functionality:

- Tracking of total staff hours (productive and paid) and total workload count for multiple reporting periods. Total hours should include agency and contracted staffing hours.
- Separate tracking of overtime and other premium pay usage.
- Calculation of productive hours per unit of service for each period.
- Calculation of required FTEs on the basis of actual workload and the target hours per UOS (budget or benchmark).
- Calculation of the FTE and cost differences between target and actual hours.
- Year-to-date or FYTD averaging for each metric.

Exhibit 13.5 is a prototype of a daily productivity report for a nursing unit. The productivity system should include executive roll-up summary reports so that senior executives can quickly review performance for all of their areas of responsibility. Senior leaders should hold their managers responsible for maintaining productivity performance and require written justification when performance is below target. Productivity monitoring data should also be used in the position control process to evaluate position requests.

Entity- and System-Level Productivity Monitoring
Productivity monitoring should also occur at the hospital or entity level. Most organizations have macro indicators to measure organizational productivity performance. Some examples of high-level productivity measures include the following:

- Total labor expense
- Total paid FTEs
- Total labor expense per case mix–adjusted equivalent discharges (CMAED)
- Total labor expense as a percentage of operating revenue
- Total paid hours and FTEs per CMAED
- Average labor cost per FTE
- Overtime as a percentage of paid hours
- Agency hours and expense

Multihospital systems frequently use these measures to benchmark overall productivity performance between their owned entities or to compare their performance with that of external institutions.

SUPPLY CHAIN VALUE ANALYSIS

The changing nature of the healthcare supply chain requires a dynamic process to continuously evaluate and manage supplies

Exhibit 13.5: Example of a Daily Productivity Report

Department: General Radiology
Units of Service: Procedures (CPT)
Average Hourly Rate: $35.60

Daily Productivity Report

Target vs. Actual Productive Hours per Unit of Service

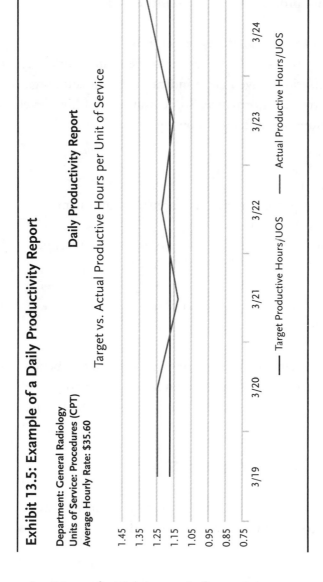

(continued)

(continued from previous page)

Exhibit 13.5: Example of a Daily Productivity Report

	3/19	3/20	3/21	3/22	3/23	3/24	3/25	Total for Period	FYTD
Units of service	259	247	256	229	258	259	201	1,709	42,725
Target productive hours	305.6	291.5	302.1	270.2	304.4	305.6	237.2	2,016.6	50,415.5
Actual productive hours	321.4	309.0	290.5	280.7	299.5	325.8	275.1	2,102.0	55,341.0
Differential actual—target	15.8	17.5	(11.6)	10.5	(4.9)	20.2	37.9	85.4	4,925.5
Actual nonproductive hours	28.9	27.8	26.5	20.3	27.0	14.2	25.0	169.7	4,242.3
Actual paid hours	350.3	336.8	317.0	301.0	326.5	340.0	300.1	2,271.7	59,583.3
Actual paid hours/UOS	1.35	1.36	1.24	1.31	1.27	1.31	1.49	1.33	1.39
Actual productive hours/UOS	1.24	1.25	1.13	1.23	1.16	1.26	1.37	1.23	1.30
Target productive hours/UOS	1.18	1.18	1.18	1.18	1.18	1.18	1.18	1.18	1.18
Differential actual—target productive hours/UOS	0.06	0.07	(0.05)	0.05	(0.02)	0.08	0.19	0.05	0.12
Productivity percentage	95.1%	94.3%	104.0%	96.3%	101.6%	93.8%	86.2%	95.9%	91.1%
Labor cost variance	$562	$624	($412)	$373	($176)	$718	$1,350	$3,040	$175,348

Note: CPT = Current Procedural Terminology; FYTD = fiscal year to date; UOS = unit of service.

and other nonlabor expenses. Many high-performing health systems institute a value analysis process to spearhead the ongoing management and improvement of medical supply expenses.

The value analysis process is driven by the work of value analysis teams (VAT). For large, multientity systems, these teams seek to achieve the following:

- Minimize the volume-adjusted supply expense for system facilities.
- Continuously evaluate and introduce high-value supplies and products to support and improve patient care.
- Provide a gatekeeping role for the introduction of new products into the system.
- Reduce variation in supply selection and usage across the organization.
- Identify and implement leading practices found within and outside the system.
- Engage physicians and clinical staff in product selection decisions.
- Consistently communicate supply issues and decisions across the system.

VAT members typically include representatives from materials management and purchasing, surgery, cardiac services, nursing, and other areas that experience high supply spending. Team members typically perform the following activities:

- Search the literature for cost-effective practices relating to medical surgical supplies.
- Act as role models to system staff in areas of value improvement and effective supply management.
- Interact with other departments to obtain user feedback on products.
- Assist in communicating and orienting system staff to changes in supply products and protocols.

- Assist with research and data collection to support product evaluations.
- Attend and participate in VAT team meetings.
- Complete all assignments for, and provide timely updates at, VAT meetings.

CASE EXAMPLE: IMPLEMENTING A VALUE ANALYSIS TEAM STRUCTURE AND PROCESS

A large multihospital health system completed an extensive operational performance improvement project to streamline costs and improve financial margins. One collaborative team focused on reducing supply and purchased services expenditures. Although the organization had a centralized materials management program, its level of standardization across the eight acute care sites was limited, particularly in regard to pharmaceutical and physician preference items.

The initial work of the collaborative team yielded more than 70 improvement initiatives with total annualized savings of $11.7 million. While the initial team results were favorable, the executive team wanted to pursue additional savings through increased product standardization and the introduction of controls over new line items brought into the system. To this end, it tasked the supply chain implementation team with developing a recommended structure and process for a systemwide VAT. Specifically, system leaders sought a VAT process that supported the following:

- Commitment to systemwide standardization of products
- Commitment to standard protocols in such areas as
  - nursing practices,
  - infection control policies, and
  - pharmacy and therapeutics (P&T) policies
- Effective communication on new-product decisions, including

- the reasons for change,
- training on the new products, and
- revised practice protocols
- Alignment with physicians on product decisions and standardization of preference items
- Ongoing measurement and management of supply usage for select categories

As a starting point, the implementation team chartered the following mission statement:

> The mission of the Value Analysis Team is to continuously seek opportunities to reduce costs and improve performance through the cost-effective selection and standardization of products, minor equipment, clinical technology and related processes, while maintaining or improving the quality of care provided to our patients.
> We believe this can best occur through:
> - Bringing together diverse perspectives
> - Challenging the status quo
> - Seeking out *leading* practices within and outside of the system
> - Focusing on maximizing health care *value*

After surveying other organizations' VAT structures and processes, the team developed the structure summarized in exhibit 13.6. In this example, the VAT team had the primary responsibilities of evaluating new product requests from physicians and staff and researching new products that have demonstrated value in other organizations. Additionally, the team evaluated and coordinated the deployment of new products introduced through the system's group purchasing programs.

The core VAT team was supported by five subteams focused on specific supply categories:

Exhibit 13.6: Value Analysis Process

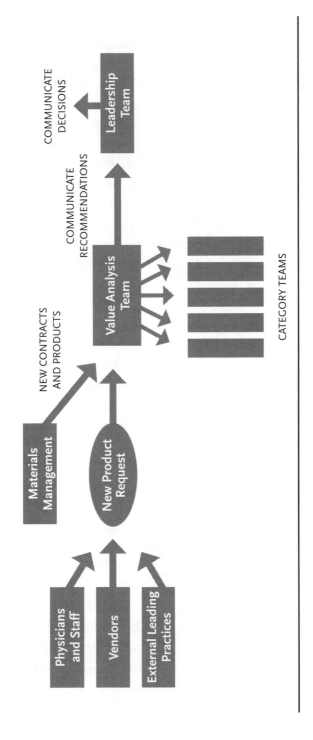

- *Medical–surgical*—reprocessing, urologicals, pulse oximetry, laundry and linen, wound care, intravenous catheters and pumps, mouth care, sharps containers
- *Perioperative supplies*—custom packs, endomechanicals, orthopedics, spine, bone and tissue, pain pumps, suction canisters, room turnover kits
- *Cardiology and radiology*—contrast media, pacemakers and implantable cardiac defibrillators, drug-eluting stents, balloons and metal stents, valves and rings
- *Laboratory*—reagents, blood products, blood collection kits, reference lab services
- *Purchased services*—transcription, nutrition, office supplies, postage and courier, forms, utilities, equipment maintenance

Pharmaceutical supply requisitions were evaluated and processed by the health system's central P&T committee.

Supply category teams were responsible for reviewing new product requests, assessing the impact of these products on the system, and providing recommendations for adoption or nonadoption to the VAT. As part of the review process, the category teams performed the following functions:

- Determined the potential economic impact (savings or cost increases) by site and for the entire system, including the new product's impact, if any, on contract compliance and tiered pricing for the product category
- Assessed the potential impact on physician preferences and satisfaction
- Gauged the impact on patients, including clinical outcomes, infection control, safety, and satisfaction
- Identified potential implementation issues, including training requirements, compatibility with other products, and materials management issues

- Assessed the potential for standardization across the system, or the potential adverse impact on product standardization, if the new item is adopted

Category teams compared the viability of the new product with the current product used (if any) and alternative substitutes. Team leaders included vendor presentations as part of the information gathered for the team to consider. The team then developed a recommendation (adopt new product, keep existing product, use an alternative product) on the basis of the option it deemed to provide the highest value to the system and its patients. For physician preference items that were rejected, the assessment included an evaluation of how the decision might affect referrals, surgery cases, and so on.

GROWTH AND STRATEGY

As part of a PI initiative, growth-oriented collaborative teams provide focus and structure for organizations to evaluate and prioritize market opportunities. Market evaluation and strategy development should be perpetual, dynamic processes for health systems to continuously evaluate the organization's growth opportunities and strategies.

Strategy and growth are often primary sources of misalignment in health systems. Many organizations operate duplicate services in geographic service areas that overlap. Often, these programs compete for the same patients and providers, and they may vary considerably by cost, patient experience, and clinical outcome.

High-performing health systems assign decision-making rights for strategy, growth, and new businesses to a system-level growth and strategy council. The growth and strategy council is led by the senior executive responsible for strategy, and members include the CEO and other executive staff, service line directors, influential physician leaders, and individuals responsible for market development.

The council performs several important functions, including the following:

- *Chart the strategic direction for the organization.* As a senior-level group, the council oversees the formation and execution of the organization's strategic initiatives. This mandate includes setting annual corporate strategic goals and growth targets. The council executes key strategic actions regarding acquisitions, partnerships, joint ventures, and other market initiatives.
- *Set expectations and oversee the work of service line leaders.* In large systems, service line executives are often challenged to implement an integrated strategy across multiple entities and markets. A growth and strategy council can make systemwide decisions and remove implementation barriers for service line leaders.
- *Make system-level decisions regarding capital and program investments.* The council prioritizes investment decisions according to determinations of what most benefits the system. This decision making includes investments in marketing, advertising, and other promotional efforts.
- *Coordinate physician recruitment and contracting.* As an important determinant of growth, the council provides strategic direction and oversight of physician recruitment. Investment decisions are made in the interest of the system and are consistent with service line needs and growth plans.
- *Oversee portfolio decisions.* The council takes the lead on portfolio decisions regarding divestment, outsourcing, building the care continuum, and similar activities.
- *Identify tactical opportunities to grow programs and revenues.* Like a growth collaborative team, the council should routinely identify and implement sales and marketing actions to grow patient volumes and net revenues.
- *Lead sales and marketing initiatives.* The council provides leadership and oversight for business development activities. As a component of this charge, the council

should continuously solicit and act on physician input regarding business development issues and opportunities.

The growth and strategy council should meet regularly, usually every two weeks. The council's agenda typically includes standing issues as well as a variety of new business. For example, the council may review such diverse issues as the following:

- Initiatives to respond to competitive inroads by a competing, misaligned physician group
- Approval of a strategic initiative to buy a local physician group
- Growth of and investment in a service line
- Strategy for how and when to take on additional risk-based contracts

KEY TAKEAWAYS FOR HIGH-IMPACT PERFORMANCE IMPROVEMENT

Today's leaders have a unique opportunity to fundamentally transform US healthcare to a value-driven system that is cost-effective and accelerates improvement in quality and outcomes for patients. However, the work required to transform healthcare systems can be daunting. Large-scale performance improvement challenges leaders at all levels of the organization and usually brings to the surface unaddressed operational, strategic, and cultural gaps. Paradoxically, leaders who are tasked with driving PI are often those individuals most threatened by the change. The fact that many transformation initiatives fall short of expectations is not surprising.

The takeaway lessons of this book are as follows:

- *Think big.* Leaders need to break from traditional, incremental improvement approaches and pursue broader, bolder interventions that hold the promise of long-term strategic and operational payoffs.
- *You don't have to start from scratch.* Most improvement opportunities in a health system can be anticipated. The key is to apply the appropriate levers to the most important areas and issues.
- *Don't wait too long to start.* This work should begin while health systems are prosperous and still evolving as integrated systems. Making long-term change is difficult for an organization that is struggling with immediate margin challenges.
- *Engage key constituents.* Leaders must align and motivate physicians, employees, and other stakeholders throughout the process or face opposition and a lack of support.
- *It's mostly about leadership.* Large-scale PI requires strong, visionary leadership from the assessment phase through implementation. Organizational change and renewal are not possible without effective executives leading the way.

Organizational Assessment Template for Performance Improvement Competencies

Performance Improvement Competency	Category	High-Performing Practice	Not in Place	Meets Some Requirements	Meets Most Requirements	Fully Meets Requirements	Notes
Performance improvement leadership	Performance improvement philosophy and approach	1. The organization has a well-defined philosophy, framework, and approach (e.g., Lean, PDCA, Six Sigma) that is uniformly understood and adopted across the organization.					
		2. The organization makes significant investments in training leaders and internal consultants on the improvement model and how it can be successfully applied to improve healthcare operations and outcomes. Certification is encouraged for persons in leadership and facilitation roles.					
		3. Knowledge and use of PI principles are evident from cultural markers such as common language, visual devices, and management routines.					
		4. The organization is adept at applying the right PI tools within the appropriate model of continuous improvement to address operational issues and drive PI. This approach is consistent across the system.					
	Performance leadership	5. Leaders consistently demonstrate knowledge of and commitment to PI through promotion of and participation in continuous improvement work.					
		6. Key leadership decisions are consistent with the espoused philosophy and culture of continuous improvement.					

Current Organizational Performance

| Performance Improvement Competency | Category | High-Performing Practice | Current Organizational Performance | | | | |
			Not in Place	Meets Some Requirements	Meets Most Requirements	Fully Meets Requirements	Notes
Performance improvement leadership		7. Senior leaders articulate and demonstrate fidelity to the model by investing personal time in the process on a regular basis.					
		8. Leaders consistently engage middle managers and staff at all levels in PI initiatives.					
	Performance improvement planning and monitoring	9. Comprehensive PI goals, with specific quantified targets, are established at least annually as part of the organization's planning process.					
		10. The organization consistently tracks progress against its improvement goals at all levels and achieves the targets it establishes.					
		11. Leaders consistently hold themselves and their team accountable for PI and adherence to operating budgets and improvement goals.					

Performance Improvement Competency	Category	High-Performing Practice		Current Organizational Performance			
			Not in Place	Meets Some Requirements	Meets Most Requirements	Fully Meets Requirements	Notes
Workforce engagement	Work culture	1. The organization has a supportive work culture that fosters collaboration and diversity consistently across the system.					
		2. Middle managers and staff feel free to share ideas and provide feedback without fear of reprisal.					
		3. The organization invests significantly in training and developing the workforce.					
	Engagement leadership	4. Senior leaders effectively communicate to all levels of the organization, particularly during a major PI initiative.					
		5. Leaders solicit staff's feedback on and involvement in PI initiatives.					
		6. Leaders consistently provide feedback to staff on performance and follow through on promises.					
		7. The organization has effective systems in place to publicly recognize and reward exceptional individual performance.					
		8. Performance reviews are tied to measurable targets that support the organization's PI goals.					
	Engagement performance	9. The organization's overall employee turnover rate is low compared to other similar healthcare organizations.					
		10. The organization's overall employee satisfaction score is in the top quartile or better when compared with other similar healthcare organizations.					

Performance Improvement Competency	Category	High-Performing Practice	Current Organizational Performance				
			Not in Place	Meets Some Requirements	Meets Most Requirements	Fully Meets Requirements	Notes
Consumer engagement	Service culture	1. The organization is adept at listening to the voice of the customer by consistently monitoring community perception and patient satisfaction through multimodal methods.					
		2. The organization defines distinct market segments and patient populations served, and it designs programs and services around the specific needs of these groups.					
		3. The organization consistently uses consumer information to identify and improve process and service gaps.					
		4. The organization routinely solicits community member feedback and input when planning new services or improving existing programs.					
		5. Clinical service leaders strive to improve quality outcomes by building patient literacy and activation.					
		6. The organization invests in programs and outreach services that build awareness and loyalty in the communities served.					
		7. The organization invests in training and scripting for associates who interface with patients and families.					
		8. The organization has highly effective procedures for follow-up on adverse service events.					
	Service outcomes	9. The organization achieves patient satisfaction scores that are in the top quartile when compared with other similar healthcare organizations.					
		10. The organization ranks as a leading provider on the basis of current community perception surveys.					

Performance Improvement Competency	Category	High-Performing Practice	Current Organizational Performance				
			Not in Place	Meets Some Requirements	Meets Most Requirements	Fully Meets Requirements	Notes
Physician engagement	Physician engagement	1. Physicians support the organization's performance initiatives.					
		2. Hospital-based physicians (e.g., pathologists, radiologists, intensivists, hospitalists, ED physicians) are engaged in productivity and performance improvement in their areas of responsibility.					
		3. Physicians are supportive of and involved with initiatives to improve patient access and throughput.					
		4. Employed physicians' incentive plans are based in part on individual and practice productivity and quality goals.					
		5. Surgeons and anesthesiologists are engaged in and aligned with surgery-related PI initiatives and supportive of efforts to improve room and staff use, room turnover, and block scheduling.					
		6. Physician executives, including the CMO, provide effective leadership as required for PI and organizational transformation to occur.					
		7. Health system leaders are effective at communicating with the medical staff (including about issues related to the organization's financial status).					
		8. Physicians generally are loyal to the organization; most referrals remain in the system, with few "splitter" physicians.					
	Physician satisfaction	9. The organization has effective systems in place to measure physician satisfaction and perceptions on a continuing basis.					
		10. The organization achieves physician satisfaction scores that are in the top quartile when compared with other similar healthcare organizations.					

Performance Improvement Competency	Category	High-Performing Practice	Current Organizational Performance				
			Not in Place	Meets Some Requirements	Meets Most Requirements	Fully Meets Requirements	Notes
Data-driven management	Key performance indicators	1. The organization uses a comprehensive, balanced set of performance metrics that accurately measure key dimensions of performance.					
		2. A layered set of KPIs tracks performance for the organization, divisions, service lines, departments, programs, and cross-functional processes.					
		3. The organization has a highly effective process in place for measuring planned versus actual performance; KPIs are tied to organizational strategic initiatives and objectives.					
		4. KPI information reflects trended data and provides comparisons against historical performance. Historical performance is provided for metrics at all levels of the organization.					
		5. The organization has an integrated system in place to report and track KPIs across performance dimensions using a dashboard capability.					
	Accessibility and competency	6. The organization has a high level of transparency with respect to KPIs; performance data are consistently shared with stakeholders, including leaders, staff, physicians, and patients.					
		7. Managers receive timely, detailed reports showing budgeted to actual expenses and revenues on at least a monthly basis. Reports show monthly and FYTD variances. Comparisons are made to the same period the previous year. Data are volume adjusted.					

Performance Improvement Competency	Category	High-Performing Practice	Current Organizational Performance				
			Not in Place	Meets Some Requirements	Meets Most Requirements	Fully Meets Requirements	Notes
Data-driven management	Performance measurement	8. Organizational leaders have a high degree of competence in performance measurement (i.e., developing metrics; understanding, analyzing, and interpreting performance data).					
		9. The organization has deep competency and highly efficient systems to support data mining and knowledge management; internal and external databases are effectively integrated.					
		10. Performance metrics and data are used consistently to identify and assign improvement teams and initiatives; these same metrics are used following implementation to determine whether improvement has been achieved.					
		11. Measurement systems are used to predict future performance and provide the basis for preemptive action—changes in strategy and tactics, contingency planning, and the automatic triggering of predefined response plans.					
		12. The organization is highly effective at identifying and integrating cause-and-effect KPIs at the departmental, process, customer segment, and organizational level.					
		13. The organization consistently uses external benchmarks across all key performance dimensions (e.g., cost, quality, productivity, service) to identify improvement opportunities and gauge performance relative to competitors.					

Note: CMO = chief medical officer; ED = emergency department; FYTD = fiscal year to date; KPI = key performance indicator; PDCA = Plan-Do-Check-Act; PI = performance improvement.

The 18 Performance Improvement Levers for Healthcare Systems

Improvement Lever	1. Process Improvement
Primary question	*What processes in the department can be simplified, eliminated, or improved in a manner that reduces resource requirements and improves customer value?*
Description	Process improvement focuses on simplifying and improving the primary tasks and services performed by a department or program. Typically, collaborative teams construct flowcharts or value maps to provide a visual depiction of how the process is currently performed. Process maps provide clarity on the sequence of steps, key inputs and outputs, and assigned roles and responsibilities.
	Next, the team evaluates points in the process that create waste, increase delays, or do not add value to customers of the work performed. Cause-and-effect analysis can also be employed to understand the presence and frequency of factors that cause a process to fail or be suboptimal.
	As improvements are identified and tested, collaborative teams construct a process map of the improved process to communicate how the process is intended to work.

Supporting tools and techniques	Process charts; value mapping; suppliers, inputs, processes, outputs, and customers (SIPOC) diagram; swim lane diagram; cause-and-effect analysis; failure mode and effects (FMEA) analysis (a methodology to reveal the myriad ways a process or system can fail or achieve adverse results); takt time analysis (takt time is the time interval required to produce one unit of service, e.g., the time to schedule an out-patient procedure); automation; muda analysis (muda represents categories of waste present in business processes)
Expected results	Simplified processes, reduced waste and redundancies, improved customer service, increased throughput and cycle time
Application examples	*Surgery:* Perioperative patient throughput, room turnover, first-case starts, instrument processing
	Laboratory: Specimen collection and processing, STAT testing, pathology results reporting
	Physician practices: Patient scheduling, patient visit throughput
	Dietary: Tray production
	Business office: Patient accounts processing

Improvement Lever	2. Structural Process Improvement
Primary question	*What key multidepartmental and cross-entity processes can be simplified, eliminated, or improved in ways that reduce resource demand while improving value to customers?*
Description	High-performing organizations are adept at applying PI initiatives to key business processes. For healthcare systems, key business processes represent those activities that have the greatest impact on patients and the provision of care. In

	an integrated health system, key processes are the primary links between system entities and ensure patients experience seamless service in their care progression.
	Key business processes are cross-functional and have scope and complexities requiring an integrative approach to improvement. Cross-functional collaborative teams typically involve a greater number of people and perspectives and require more time to complete process change than a functional-level collaborative team requires.
Supporting tools and techniques	Process charts, value mapping, SIPOC diagram, swim lane diagram, cause-and-effect analysis, FMEA analysis, takt time analysis, automation, muda analysis, automation, kaizen planning
Expected results	Improved, seamless service for patients, lowered operating expenses, reduction in errors associated with hand-offs between functional areas
Application examples	*Ambulatory care:* Patient access and scheduling, referrals to specialists and hospital services, professional billing, outpatient service delivery *Acute care:* Patient admissions and preadmissions processes, perioperative throughput, emergency department patient throughput, outpatient scheduling and registration, bed control and room turnover, supply chain management, patient discharge processes, patient charging and billing *Post-acute care:* Acute case transfers to post-acute providers, home care service delivery, patient charging and billing

Improvement Lever	3. Facility Optimization
Primary question	*Are improvements to be made to the layout and workspace of our department that will improve patient flow and facilitate effective use of our resources?*
Description	The layout and design of a department or facility can have a significant impact on staff productivity and the flow of patients, equipment, and supplies. Staff productivity can be adversely affected by facilities that result in the following: • Increased travel and patient transport time • Increased time searching for supplies and equipment • Lack of space to perform work or to collaborate with other staff • Lack of capacity to accommodate additional cases, resulting in idle staff and potential loss of revenues • Poor patient throughput, resulting in delays and nonvalue work Facility design can also pertain to the design and condition of an individual's workspace or a small department work area. Managers should ensure that all work areas are clean, orderly, and safe for patients and staff.
Supporting tools and techniques	Five S analysis, simulation, physical process maps, spaghetti diagrams, proximity charting
Expected results	Reduced non-value-added time for travel and other staff time, improved inventory and equipment management, improved safety and security, improved patient throughput

Application examples	*Emergency services*: Capacity management and patient flow
	Surgery: Operating room (OR) capacity and patient flow between perioperative services
	Sterile processing: Layout and flow of processing area for equipment sterilization
	Labor and delivery: Integrated facility design for prenatal, delivery, and postpartum services

Improvement Lever	4. Demand Smoothing
Primary question	*How can we schedule patients and work activities in a way that balances workload across the day and the week?*
Description	Maintaining high performance is facilitated when workload is evenly distributed throughout the day and the week. To this end, managers should implement demand-smoothing strategies to reduce workload variation commensurate with their ability to control demand.
	The two primary components of demand smoothing are as follows:
	Patient scheduling. Leaders should schedule nonemergency, elective patient cases and visits in a manner that minimizes daily and weekly workload variation. Such scheduling often involves working with physicians who influence the timing of patient care tasks.
	Work scheduling. Nonurgent work assignments and tasks (i.e., deferrable work) should be scheduled when patient demand is low.
Supporting tools and techniques	Demand profiling, demand segmentation, task analysis (identify deferrable tasks), heijunka (a method to level out production in a way that reduces waste and achieves flexible, predictable, and stable outcomes; also defined as level scheduling)

Expected results	Increased productivity, improved quality and safety, reduction in errors and rework, reduced wait times, improved customer service and satisfaction
Application examples	*Case management*: Working with physicians to complete discharge orders earlier in the day than usual
	Surgery: Using block scheduling to evenly distribute surgery cases throughout the day and the week
	Information services: Scheduling technology conversions and installations during off hours to minimize the impact on users
	Physician practices: Scheduling a balanced mix of visit types (e.g., routine visits, follow-up visits, new patient evaluations) to balance workload throughout the week

Improvement Lever	5. Demand Regrouping
Primary question	*Can we reaggregate work in ways that will improve alignment of resources, build proficiencies, and enhance workload balancing?*
Description	Demand regrouping represents the myriad possibilities of grouping work tasks to improve efficiencies and effectiveness.
	Benefits to grouping common work include the following:
	• Allows enhanced alignment of staffing and skill mix to the work requirement
	• Creates a critical mass of like tasks and skill requirements, enabling assigned staff to develop their proficiency and improve the quality of the work performed
	• Can improve equipment and facility utilization

	The following regrouping strategies are applicable to healthcare delivery:
	Patient aggregation. Performance improvement (PI) initiatives should consider opportunities to regroup work. Two primary strategies for patient grouping are
	• patient-needs based, whereby patients are grouped primarily according to their total care needs or acuity, and • service based, whereby patients are grouped on the basis of service line designation or by physician group.
	System-level aggregation. Patients with specific service needs and diagnoses are directed to a single, central location in a regional system. This type of aggregation is often a result of clinical rationalization and the development of centers of excellence that have a specific clinical area of focus.
	Nonclinical regrouping. The concept of work regrouping is equally applicable in nonclinical areas, such as the business office, sterile processing, and case management.
Supporting tools and techniques	Demand segmentation, activity analysis, workload forecasting, and predictive analytics
Expected results	Improved quality and performance, improved staff proficiency, lowered costs as a result of pooling subscale services
Application examples	*Acute care nursing:* Assigning patients to units on the basis of similar needs *Pediatrics:* Creating a single pediatric inpatient program for a multihospital system *Business office:* Organizing work on the basis of payer group *Emergency services:* Grouping patients by severity or primary diagnosis

Improvement Lever	6. Role and Team Redesign
Primary question	*How can we design roles and assign responsibilities in a way that will achieve improved flexibility and workload balance across our staff?*
Description	Leaders should pursue role and team redesign with the following collective goals: • Enhancing service provision for patients and other internal and external customers • Increasing the flexibility of labor resources to respond to changing workload demand • Reducing redundant and non-value-added work • Continuously improving the skills and proficiency of the workforce • Developing roles that provide challenge and fulfillment for staff Effective role and team redesign must achieve a balance of three primary goals: • *Balanced workload.* Each staff member should have a reasonable and comparable share of the workload. • *Shared workload.* Staff should be cross-trained so tasks (those without licensure restrictions) can be shared in and across job classes. • *Challenging work.* Job design should ensure that all roles include responsibilities that are rewarding and leverage an individual's skills, training, and abilities. Role design is a critical factor in the organization's ability to match staffing resources to demand and to provide responsive service to patients and physicians. Role design also has a significant impact on staff satisfaction and the costs and issues resulting from employee turnover.

Supporting tools and techniques	Activity analysis, standardized work, work balancing, training and development
Expected results	Increased productivity, improved quality and safety, improved customer service, enhanced staff satisfaction
Application examples	*Support services*: Multiskilled, unit-assigned service associate role
	Medical imaging: Training technologists in multiple modalities
	Nursing services: Patient care team design and role delineation for licensed and nonlicensed staff
	Surgical services: Delineation of tasks and responsibilities by skill level for OR room turnover

Improvement Lever	7. Dynamic Staffing
Primary question	*What strategies can we employ to ensure that we have sufficient staffing to meet variable workload demand?*
Description	High-performing healthcare organizations proactively employ flexible staffing strategies to meet changes in workload volumes. These strategies enable leaders to quickly deploy staffing resources across departments and system entities when volumes are high. Other strategies enable organizations to decrease capacity when demand falls. Flexible staffing includes the following categories:
	Central float pools. Staffing pools are useful, whether used in a single organization or across multiple system entities, to provide daily coverage and surge capacity. The most common application of float pools in healthcare is for acute care nurse staffing. Many hospitals employ nursing float pools to allocate staffing resources across multiple inpatient units.

	System float pools. Regional multihospital systems can also implement float pools to share staffing of skilled technical roles, including pharmacists, surgical nurses, imaging technologists, laboratory technologists, and physical and occupational therapists. Regional float pools are limited by geographic distance and location. *Seasonal staffing strategies.* Many healthcare systems experience seasonal spikes in workload that require the use of short-term staffing and premium pay allowance to provide sufficient staffing capacity. *Contingency staffing plans.* Healthcare providers should institute plans that reassign staffing in a shift as dictated by throughput backlogs and other conditions.
Supporting tools and techniques	Demand profiling, demand segmentation, workload forecasting and predictive analytics, training and development
Expected results	Increased productivity, improved quality and safety, reduction in errors and rework, reduced wait times, improved customer service and satisfaction
Application examples	*Acute care*: Centralized float pool for registered nurses and unlicensed staff *Imaging, rehabilitation therapy, pharmacy*: System-level float pools *Emergency services*: Contingency staffing strategies *All departments*: Low-census and seasonality plans defined by cost center

Improvement Lever	8. Management Restructuring
Primary question	*Are opportunities available to leverage executive or management roles across departments, programs, and sites?*
Description	PI initiatives typically include an evaluation of the leadership structure with the goal of reducing management layers and redundancies. Management restructuring should begin with a span-of-control analysis, which inventories all leadership positions and records the number of direct reports for each management position. The continuing consolidation of hospitals into large regional systems presents additional opportunities for organizations to leverage and streamline management resources across multiple entities. Management restructuring frequently occurs early in the development of a healthcare system. In addition to reducing labor expense, a consolidated leadership team is better positioned to drive postmerger program and operational consolidation. Regional leadership decisions fall somewhere on a continuum between a totally centralized model and a totally decentralized model as described next: • *Centralized.* Most or all leadership is consolidated to the regional level, with limited leadership retained at the site level. • *Decentralized.* Leadership is required at each site; few opportunities are available to centralize. • *Partially centralized.* A mix of centralized and decentralized leaders; for example, subregional responsibilities are assigned so that leadership is spread over 2 or 3 sites on the basis of proximity or other factors.

Supporting tools and techniques	Span-of-control analysis, leadership development, role design, team building
Expected results	Lowered labor expense, increased leadership consistency across the system, reduced levels of management, increased span of control
Application examples	Most administrative services Clinical service line leadership Leadership for support and other centralized and corporate services

Improvement Lever	9. System Rationalization
Primary question	*Are opportunities available to consolidate duplicate programs at the system or corporate levels?*
Description	System rationalization is the process by which health systems identify opportunities to consolidate duplicate programs and services with the following goals: • Driving down operating costs by eliminating fixed expenses • Repositioning services and programs in the market to improve the organization's competitive position • Consolidating demand across small, subscale programs • Maintaining or improving access and services to patients and internal customers of the system Rationalized cost savings can accrue from several sources, depending on the function. Sources include the following: • Consolidating management staffing • Rationalizing administrative support positions • Rationalizing specialist staff • Batching workload at a central site to lower cost per unit

	• Reducing purchased services • Reducing duplicate supply inventories • Reducing duplicate facilities, rent, and capital equipment
Supporting tools and techniques	Activity-based costing, return-on-investment (ROI) analysis, market assessment
Expected results	Reduced operating expenses, enhanced service coordination across markets, standardization of processes and system protocols
Application examples	*Administrative services*: Human resources, marketing, administration, training and development *Clinical services*: Consolidation of select services *Centralized services*: Laboratory, business office

Improvement Lever	10. Service Redeployment
Primary question	*Should we should physically relocate any staff resources or services to a different area to improve service and lower operating costs?*
Description	Cross-functional process design frequently requires decisions to be made concerning service redeployment. Service redeployment is the physical relocation of staff, equipment, and other resources close to where services are most needed. Locating resources at the point of demand can yield several organizational benefits: • Improved service response time for patients and internal customers • Reduced travel time for staff • Reduced patient transportation time • Reduced service scheduling and coordination for caregivers and other staff • Increased opportunities for developing multiskilled roles

	• Increased opportunities to rationalize management resources Service redeployment can occur on a small, intradepartmental basis, among several departments, or across health system entities and markets.
Supporting tools and techniques	Value mapping, physical process maps, spaghetti diagrams, proximity charting, activity analysis
Expected results	Improved customer response time, improved staff utilization, reduced labor expense
Application examples	*Laboratory*: Redeploying phlebotomy responsibilities to nursing unit–based staff *Accounting*: Redeploying centralized controller positions to entities to improve service responsiveness *Patient transportation*: Assigning centralized transport staff to high-volume patient care service areas *Respiratory therapy*: Assigning routine respiratory therapy procedures to patient care staff

Improvement Lever	11. Nonlabor Optimization
Primary question	***Are improvements to our supply chain processes and other nonlabor expenses available that will reduce staff time and lower spending on supplies, equipment, and purchased services?***
Description	Clinical care requires significant use of supplies and equipment. Consequently, clinicians can spend considerable time in supply-related activities, including managing inventory, searching for supplies and equipment, cleaning and sterilization of equipment, and charging for supplies usage. Excessive inventories increase holding costs and require additional staff for supply receiving, storage, and distribution.

	Healthcare managers should focus on supply strategies that accomplish the following:
	• Simplify and improve supply chain processes to minimize time requirements for clinical staff
	• Locate high-usage supply items at the point of care to minimize clinical staff time spent searching for needed items
	• Leverage technology to simplify supply inventory management and patient charging
	• Minimize on-hand inventories that drive up holding costs and materials management staffing
	• Maintain patient care equipment to minimize equipment malfunction and delays in patient care caused by missing equipment
	Similarly, leaders should evaluate purchased services and other nonlabor expenditures to identify improvement opportunities.
Supporting tools and techniques	Kanban (a Lean scheduling improvement technique that minimizes inventories at all points of production) and pull systems, physical process maps, overall equipment effectiveness, just-in-time (JIT) inventory, point-of-use storage
Expected results	Reduced non-value-added time for travel and other staff time, improved inventory and equipment management
Application examples	*Cardiac services*: Reduce costs of cardiac implants through improved pricing and demand management

Materials management: Reduce holding costs through JIT and consignment inventory

Nursing: Increase the time between change-outs for IVs to reduce utilization |

	Purchased services: Legal and consulting expenses, maintenance contracts, travel expenditures, professional services contracts, utilities

Improvement Lever	12. Off-Quality Improvement
Primary question	*What areas of clinical and service quality performance can be improved that will have the most significant impact on outcomes and operating costs?*
Description	Adverse quality and safety events add considerable costs to patient care services. Organizations need effective surveillance systems to monitor quality and safety performance, by case and by physician. As off-quality events occur, the organization must have effective protocols in place for engaging physicians and improving performance.
	Improving quality can have a direct financial impact on costs and reimbursement. The advent of value-based purchasing (VBP) and penalties for readmissions means that payers will no longer reimburse low-quality and unnecessary utilization. Population health incentives will further require healthcare providers to focus on quality improvement and reducing the incidence of off-quality events.
	Service quality performance is critical for maintaining high levels of patient satisfaction. Low patient satisfaction can result in market share decline and reduced operating revenues.
Supporting tools and techniques	Measurement systems for clinical quality performance, patient satisfaction surveys, costing systems to measure the financial impact of off-quality events

Expected results	Improved quality outcomes, cost avoidance, increased revenues, improved patient satisfaction
Application examples	*Patient safety*: Reduction in off-quality clinical events
	Revenue cycle: Increased VBP reimbursement, reduction in denials
	Patient satisfaction: Increased patient satisfaction and customer retention

Improvement Lever	13. Clinical Utilization Improvement
Primary question	*Are opportunities available to reduce unnecessary utilization of services that will in turn reduce the cost of care while maintaining or improving outcomes?*
Description	Utilization management represents myriad improvement strategies employed by healthcare organizations to reduce unnecessary or low-value workload. Nowhere is utilization management more evident than in the provision of patient care services. In most healthcare systems, significant opportunities are available to decrease healthcare costs by reducing clinically unnecessary or redundant testing or procedures and by improving quality and patient safety.
	Reducing acute care service costs represents a significant opportunity for most provider organizations. The advents of population health and accountable care require hospitals to evaluate and improve acute care cost performance. Payment methodologies for Medicare and most other payers have shifted to a per case or per diem basis. Many organizations have instituted bundled pricing strategies that combine the hospital and physician costs into a fixed, all-inclusive price for payers. As a result, any overutilization of care reduces the per case contribution margin for patient care.

	Utilization management principles can apply to any work environment where opportunities exist to eliminate or reduce nonvalue work.
Supporting tools and techniques	Demand profiling, activity-based costing, clinical benchmarking
Expected results	Lowered cost per case, increased contribution margins, improved patient throughput, potential improvements to outcomes and patient safety
Application examples	*Orthopedics*: Demand matching for orthopedic implants *Labor and delivery*: Reduction in cesarean-section rates *Nursing services*: Reduction in length of stay for acute care patients *All departments*: Reduction in non-value-added work

Improvement Lever	14. Demand Growth
Primary question	*Do we anticipate short-term growth in this department that will result in higher staff utilization?*
Description	Performance management plans need to include strategies for achieving market share and revenue growth. Healthcare organizations must achieve growth in services that generate sufficient contribution margin to cover overhead expenses. With the advent of accountable care, providers increasingly will be paid on an at-risk basis. Health systems will seek to grow revenues by managing the health of defined patient populations. The transition from fee-for-service to accountable care will require organizations to pursue growth opportunities in both markets.

	Growth initiatives typically focus on short-term, tactical opportunities to increase patient volumes and revenues. Tactical growth can occur in several ways, including the following:
	<ul><li>Reducing leakage of referrals from affiliated physicians</li><li>Creating new demand through improved diagnosis of patient conditions and referral to the appropriate service or clinician</li><li>Freeing capacity in surgery and other clinical departments to reduce case backlogs</li><li>Shifting providers and resources to build capacity in growing markets</li></ul> Other growth strategies take longer than those listed above; however, they may be included in the scope of a growth-oriented collaborative team. Examples of long-term growth initiatives include the following: <ul><li>Recruiting new physicians to increase patient referrals and procedures</li><li>Building new programs and care sites to pursue new markets</li><li>Purchasing other provider organizations</li><li>Launching new joint ventures with other providers</li></ul>
Supporting tools and techniques	Market assessment, competitor analysis, profit-and-loss (P&L) analysis of current programs
Expected results	Market share and revenue growth, improved success rate of new business ventures, improved productivity resulting from overall workload increases
Application examples	Growth principles are applicable to any service with patient revenues, but they are most frequently applied to high-margin outpatient and ambulatory services.

Improvement Lever	15. Revenue Optimization
Primary question	*What changes can we make in the revenue cycle that will increase net revenues?*
Description	Today's revenue cycle is multidisciplinary in scope and demands a high level of functional integration and collaboration within the organization. Reimbursement from payers continues to decrease as payment responsibility shifts to consumers via increased deductibles and copayments. This reduction of third-party reimbursement creates the potential for significant bad debt and cash lag issues if not well managed.

PI initiatives should include a focus on revenue cycle improvements. Improvements to the revenue cycle accrue directly to an organization's top-line revenues and operating margin.

Improvement initiatives should consider all components of the revenue cycle, including those discussed next:

- *Preservice.* Pricing, contracting, preregistration, scheduling, insurance verification, preauthorization, financial clearance, financial responsibility and collection, visitor education
- *Point of service (POS).* Referrals, stop gaps, charge capture, POS collections, coding, clinical documentation
- *Postservice.* Payer management, bad debt management, accounts receivable (A/R) follow-up with patient, A/R follow-up with payer, payment posting, denial management, expected payment calculation, claims processing, charge reconciliation |
| **Supporting tools and techniques** | Process improvement, value mapping, automation, benchmarking, standard work design |

Expected results	Increased net revenues, reduced denials, improved A/R metrics, lowered bad debt
Application examples	*Materials management*: Implementing automated supply dispensing to improve charge capture
	Clinical documentation: Working with physicians to improve documentation and coding and reduce denials
	Patient registration: Increasing POS collections
	Finance: Improving terms by and reimbursement from commercial insurance providers

Improvement Lever	16. Service Outsourcing
Primary question	**Can outsourcing improve the cost and service performance of a department or program?**
Description	Organizations often perform services and functions that are necessary to their business, but they do not have the resources or experience to deliver those services in an optimal manner. Outsourcing represents the "buy" option in the make-versus-buy improvement determination of portfolio management. Many organizations source programs and functions to external companies that have the expertise and focus to provide the service more effectively than the healthcare systems can.
	Outsourcing is a common strategy employed by organizations to reduce operating expenses, particularly in noncore, support, and administrative services. Cost saving is not the only driver of outsourcing decisions.
	Organizations also outsource services to other firms for the following reasons:
	• Improve organizational focus on core services

	• Gain access to best practices and technologies • Obtain expertise and management talent that is difficult to attract and retain • Free up internal resources and capital for redeployment to other priorities • Share financial risk • Provide investment and cash infusion
Supporting tools and techniques	Activity-based costing, ROI analysis, benchmarking, customer surveys
Expected results	Lowered costs, maintained or improved service, improved focus on core services
Application examples	*Laboratory*: Outsourcing specialty testing to a reference laboratory *Support services*: Outsourcing services to an outside vendor *Transcription*: Outsourcing transcription services to a freelance transcriber *Marketing and public relations*: Hire contractors for writing, photography, web development, and other select services

Improvement Lever	17. Service Divestment
Primary question	*What programs and services should we consider discontinuing?*
Description	For some programs, services, or entities, the best improvement option may be to shut down or sell the service to another organization. For health systems, service divestment usually occurs with patient care services, community programs, grant-funded initiatives, or facilities that no longer fit effectively with the organization's portfolio. Frequently, these decisions are precipitated by changing market conditions or economic issues, as with the following scenarios:

	• An outreach program has lost the funding that had sustained it in the past. • A joint venture with a physician's group has been dissolved. • An outpatient surgery facility is closed after having struggled for years to break even in a highly competitive market. • A hospital decides to close a child care center due to underutilization. • A multihospital system sells one of its hospitals to invest in a different market. • A program that is struggling to build patient volumes experiences declining revenues and limited opportunities for incremental productivity improvement. Service divestment decisions are rarely easy to implement. Eliminating programs and services can negatively affect patients and staff. Health-care leaders must anticipate the impact of these decisions on constituent groups, communicate the changes and the reasons for the decision, and provide service alternatives. Expected cost savings must be balanced with implementation costs, such as severance pay, lost revenues, and legal expenses.
Supporting tools and techniques	Activity-based costing, ROI analysis, benchmarking, customer surveys, and customer impact assessment
Expected results	Lowered costs, maintained or improved service (if the service is assumed by a qualified provider), improved focus on core services
Application examples	Service divestment can apply to most noncore services.

Improvement Lever	18. Continuum Realignment
Primary question	*How should we realign resources and invest-ments across the care continuum in response to market changes?*
Description	Healthcare delivery shifts and reimbursement reform are changing how care is organized and provided in the United States. Healthcare systems in turn are being transformed by the following: • A shift from acute care to ambulatory care • An increase in rehabilitation and post-acute services • An increase in home-based care supported by telemedicine technology • An increase in procedures performed in physician offices and other ambulatory settings • An increase in population health • Growth in risk-based contracting and provider-sponsored health plans Continuum realignment represents the myriad strategies employed by health systems to transi-tion operations from a predominantly acute care model to an integrated care system encom-passing multiple components of care delivery. Continuum realignment determines the stra-tegic decisions regarding investments in new programs and disinvestment in others. The end goal is to retool the healthcare system to build population health capabilities and sup-port accountable care. Continuum realignment is a long-term improvement lever, but it has the potential to transform healthcare provider organizations.
Supporting tools and techniques	Market demand assessment, competitor analysis, P&L analysis of current programs and services, actuarial risk analysis

Expected results	New service capabilities, integrated care delivery, population health
Application examples	*Physician practices*: Building a primary care network of physician practices through acquisition and joint ventures
	Home care: Implementing a patient-centered medical home model for home-based care delivery
	Population health: Contracting with insurance providers to operate under an at-risk payment model for a defined patient population
	Acute care: Downsizing acute care capacity as more care shifts to ambulatory settings

Application of Improvement Levers by Functional Area

Function	Improving Processes and Facilities				Aligning Resources with Demand				Leveraging the System			Optimizing Nonlabor	Improving Quality and Utilization		Building Top-Line Revenues		Optimizing the Service Portfolio		
	1. Process Improvement	2. Structural Process Improvement	3. Facility Optimization	4. Demand Smoothing	5. Demand Regrouping	6. Role and Team Redesign	7. Dynamic Staffing	8. Management Restructuring	9. System Rationalization	10. Service Redeployment	11. Nonlabor Optimization	12. Off-Quality Improvement	13. Utilization Management	14. Demand Growth	15. Revenue Optimization	16. Service Outsourcing	17. Service Divestment	18. Continuum Realignment
Accounting	▨	▨			▨	▨		■		▨								
Administrative services								■									■	▨
Admissions and registration	■	■	■	■		▨	■	▨	▨	▨		▨				▨		
Anesthesia	▨	▨		▨						▨		▨	▨					
Biomedical engineering		▨							■			▨				■		
Business office/ patient accounts	■	▨		▨	▨	■	▨	■	■					■				
Cardiac cath lab	▨			■		▨				■		▨	▨	■		▨		▨
Cardiac rehab	▨			■			▨							▨		▨		
Case management		▨	▨		▨	▨			▨		■	■				▨		
CT scan	▨	▨	▨	▨		▨	■			▨		▨	■	▨				
Dialysis	▨	▨		■			▨					▨	▨		■	■		
Dietary services	■	■	■			▨	▨									▨		
EKG/EEG		▨			■				■				▨		▨			

Function	Improving Processes and Facilities			Aligning Resources with Demand				Leveraging the System			Optimizing Nonlabor	Improving Quality and Utilization		Building Top-Line Revenues		Optimizing the Service Portfolio		
	1. Process Improvement	2. Structural Process Improvement	3. Facility Optimization	4. Demand Smoothing	5. Demand Regrouping	6. Role and Team Redesign	7. Dynamic Staffing	8. Management Restructuring	9. System Rationalization	10. Service Redeployment	11. Nonlabor Optimization	12. Off-Quality Improvement	13. Utilization Management	14. Demand Growth	15. Revenue Optimization	16. Service Outsourcing	17. Service Divestment	18. Continuum Realignment
Emergency services																		
Endoscopy/GI lab																		
Foundation																		
Health information/medical records																		
Home health services																		
Housekeeping/environmental services																		
Human resources																		
ICU/CCU																		
Infection control																		
IT																		
Labor and delivery																		
Laboratory																		

Note: cath = catheterization; CCU = critical care unit; CT = computed tomography; EEG = electroencephalogram; EKG = electrocardiogram; GI = gastrointestinal; ICU = intensive care unit; IT = information technology.

References

Ackoff, R. L., J. Magidson, and H. J. Addison. 2006. *Idealized Design: Creating an Organization's Future.* Upper Saddle River, NJ: Prentice-Hall.

Agency for Healthcare Research and Quality (AHRQ). 2017. "Transforming the Organization and Delivery of Primary Care." Accessed August 23. www.pcmh.ahrq.gov.

Berwick, D. M., T. W. Nolan, and J. Whittington. 2008. "The Triple Aim: Care, Health, and Cost." *Health Affairs* 27 (3): 759–69.

Centers for Medicare & Medicaid Services (CMS). 2017a. "Accountable Care Organizations (ACO)." Updated May 12. www.cms.gov/Medicare/Medicare-Fee-for-Service-Payment/ACO/index.html?redirect=/aco.

———. 2017b. "Core Measures." Updated July 28. www.cms.gov/Medicare/Quality-initiatives-patient-assessment-instruments/quality measures/core-measures.html.

———. 2017c. "Readmissions Reduction Program (HRRP)." Updated November 30. www.cms.gov/medicare/medicare-fee-for-service-payment/acuteinpatientpps/readmissions-reduction-program.html.

———. 2017d. "What Are the Value-Based Programs?" Updated November 9. www.cms.gov/Medicare/Quality-Initiatives-Patient-Assessment-Instruments/Value-Based-Programs/Value-Based-Programs.html.

———. 2014. "HCAHPS: Patients' Perspectives of Care Survey." Updated September 25. www.cms.gov/Medicare/Quality-Initiatives

-Patient-Assessment-Instruments/HospitalQualityInits/Hospital
HCAHPS.html.

Chalfin, D. B., S. Trzeciak, A. Likourezos, B. M. Baumann, and R.
P. Dellinger. 2007. "Impact of Delayed Transfer of Critically Ill
Patients from the Emergency Department to the Intensive Care
Unit." *Critical Care Medicine* 35 (6): 1477–83.

Chalice, R. 2007. *Improving Healthcare Using Toyota Lean Production
Methods: 46 Steps for Improvement.* Milwaukee, WI: ASQ Quality
Press.

Coffey, R. J. 2005. "Engineering and the Health Care System." In
*Building a Better Delivery System: A New Engineering/Health Care
Partnership*, edited by P. P. Reid, W. D. Compton, J. H. Grossman,
and G. Fanjiang, 107–11. Washington, DC: National Academies
Press.

Crosby, P. B. 1986. *Quality Is Free: The Art of Making Quality Certain.*
New York: McGraw-Hill.

Dean, M. L. 2013. *Lean Healthcare Deployment and Sustainability.* New
York: McGraw-Hill Education.

Deming, W. E. 1986. *Out of the Crisis.* Cambridge, MA: Center
for Advanced Engineering Study, Massachusetts Institute of
Technology.

Emanuel, E. J., and V. R. Fuchs. 2008. "The Perfect Storm of Overutilization." *Journal of the American Medical Association* 299 (23):
2789–91.

Graban, M., and J. E. Swartz. 2014. *The Executive Guide to Healthcare Kaizen: Leadership for a Continuously Learning and Improving
Organization.* Boca Raton, FL: CRC Press.

Hammer, M. 1990. "Reengineering Work: Don't Automate, Obliter-
ate." *Harvard Business Review* 9 (4): 104–13.

Herzlinger, R. 1997. *Market-Driven Health Care: Who Wins, Who
Loses in the Transformation of America's Largest Service Industry.*
Cambridge, MA: Perseus.

Hibbard, J. H., and J. Greene. 2013. "What the Evidence Shows About
Patient Activation: Better Health Outcomes and Care Experiences;
Fewer Data on Costs." *Health Affairs* 32 (2): 207–14.

Institute of Medicine. 2001. *Crossing the Quality Chasm: A New Health System for the 21st Century*. Washington, DC: National Academies Press.

Juran, J. M. 1989. *Juran on Leadership for Quality: An Executive Handbook*. New York: Free Press.

Kane, M., K. Chui, J. Rimicci, P. Callagy, J. Hereford, S. Shen, R. Norris, and D. Pickham. 2015. "Lean Manufacturing Improves Emergency Department Throughput and Patient Satisfaction." *Journal of Nursing Administration* 45 (9): 429–34.

Kripalani, S., C. N. Theobald, B. Anctil, and E. E. Vasilevskis. 2014. "Reducing Hospital Readmission Rates: Current Strategies and Future Directions." *Annual Review of Medicine* 65: 471–85.

Larson, J. A. 2014. *Management Engineering: A Guide to Best Practices for Industrial Engineering in Health Care*. New York: CRC Press.

Lathrop, J. P. 1993. *Restructuring Health Care: The Patient Focused Paradigm*. San Francisco: Jossey-Bass.

Leander, W. J. 1996. *Patients First: Experiences of a Patient-Focused Pioneer*. Chicago: Health Administration Press.

Leebov, W., and C. J. Ersoz. 2003. *The Health Care Manager's Guide to Continuous Quality Improvement*. New York: Authors Choice Press.

Manion, J., W. Lorimer, and W. J. Leander. 1996. *Team-Based Health Care Organizations: Blueprint for Success*. Gaithersburg, MD: Aspen.

Medicare.gov. 2017. "Find a Hospital." Accessed August 23. www.medicare.gov/hospitalcompare/search.html.

Miles, R. H. 2010. "Accelerating Corporate Transformations—Don't Lose Your Nerve!" *Harvard Business Review* (January–February): 68–75.

National Institute of Standards and Technology (NIST). 2017. "Baldrige Performance Excellence Program." Accessed December 18. www.nist.gov/baldrige.

NORC at the University of Chicago. 2016. "Trends in Hospital Inpatient Drug Costs: Issues and Challenges." Published October 11. www.aha.org/content/16/aha-fah-rx-report.pdf.

Parker, B. T., and C. Marco. 2014. "Emergency Department Length of Stay: Accuracy of Patient Estimates." *Western Journal of Emergency Medicine* 15 (2): 170–75.

Porter, M. E., and E. O. Teisberg. 2006. *Redefining Health Care: Creating Value-Based Competition on Results.* Boston: Harvard Business School Press.

Reider, R. 2000. *Benchmarking Strategies: A Tool for Profit Improvement.* New York: Wiley.

Singer, A. J., H. C. Thode, P. Viccellio, and J. M. Pines. 2011. "The Association Between Length of Emergency Department Boarding and Mortality." *Academic Emergency Medicine* 18 (12): 1324–29.

Smalley, H. E. 1982. *Hospital Management Engineering: A Guide to the Improvement of Hospital Management Systems.* Englewood Cliffs, NJ: Prentice-Hall.

Tague, N. R. 2005. "Pareto Chart." In *The Quality Toolbox*, 2nd ed., 376–78. Milwaukee, WI: ASQ Quality Press.

Tsai, T. C., J. E. Oray, and A. K. Jha. 2015. "Patient Satisfaction and Quality of Surgical Care in US Hospitals." *Annals of Surgery* 261 (1): 2–8.

Wedgwood, I. D. 2007. *Lean Sigma: A Practitioner's Guide.* Upper Saddle River, NJ: Prentice-Hall.

About the Author

Gary M. Auton is a senior director with Galloway Consulting, based in Atlanta. He has more than 30 years of consulting experience providing strategic and operational advisory services to a broad range of private- and public-sector organizations, including hospitals, health plans, physician practices, employer health coalitions, and state and federal health agencies. Previous clients include more than 150 hospitals and health systems located throughout the United States and internationally. He served on the board of examiners of the National Institute of Standards and Technology's Baldrige Performance Excellence Program.

Auton has a bachelor of science degree in health systems from the Georgia Institute of Technology and an MBA with a concentration in strategic management and entrepreneurship from Georgia State University. He is Lean Six Sigma Green Belt certified through the University of Michigan College of Engineering's Integrative Systems and Design certification program. Auton is a frequent speaker at healthcare conferences and was a featured healthcare writer for *Competitive Edge* business magazine.

ABOUT GALLOWAY CONSULTING

Galloway Consulting, a subsidiary of ADAMS Management Services Corporation, is an Atlanta-based professional advisory firm serving the healthcare industry. For the past 20 years, Galloway has helped more than 450 clients, including academic medical centers, national and regional health systems, and individual facilities, improve operations, outcomes, and profits. The Galloway consulting team brings together decades of professional experience in healthcare consulting, hospital management, medical group management, corporate consulting, and IT system implementation.

Representative Galloway projects include engagements focused on growth, organization design, governance improvement, portfolio analysis, program development, operations improvement, quality and service improvement, leadership coaching, performance measurement, and change initiative implementation.